Manual for Night-Time Emergencies for Pediatric Hematology-Oncology Fellows

Being on call as a pediatric resident or a pediatric hematology-oncology fellow can cause great anxiety. In addition to the relatively common patient with chemotherapy-related fever and neutropenia, there is the anticipation of problems that a trainee may have read about but not yet actually seen—the adolescent newly presenting with a white blood cell count of 600,000/mm^3, the 2-year-old spitting up blood with a platelet count of 2,000/ mm^3 and a hemoglobin of 5g/dL, the child who comes to the ER with difficulty walking and is found to have a paraspinal mass on MRI. Most issues can wait until the next day when more senior practitioners are around, but some are true medical emergencies and just can't.

This manual is intended as a one-stop solution for such frantic moments—a quick resource to bridge the hours between the start of night call and morning rounds that focuses on what needs to be done immediately to avoid hurting a patient. It offers succinct guidelines and algorithms to address the emergencies most likely to come up overnight. For those tempted to turn to AI for quick solutions, there are some salutary lessons from responses AI has given when asked about such emergencies.

Manual for Night-Time Emergencies for Pediatric Hematology-Oncology Fellows
Should We Chat?

Julie Blatt MD

Division of Pediatric Hematology-Oncology,
The University of North Carolina at Chapel Hill, NC

April M. Evans MD MPH

Department of Hematology-Oncology,
Roger Maris Cancer Center, Fargo, ND

Jessica Benjamin-Eze DO

Division of Pediatric Hematology-Oncology,
The University of North Carolina at Chapel Hill, NC

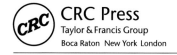

CRC Press
Taylor & Francis Group
Boca Raton New York London

CRC Press is an imprint of the
Taylor & Francis Group, an **informa** business

Designed cover image: Shutterstock and Gerardo Quezada

First edition published 2025
by CRC Press
2385 NW Executive Center Drive, Suite 320, Boca Raton FL 33431

and by CRC Press
4 Park Square, Milton Park, Abingdon, Oxon, OX14 4RN

CRC Press is an imprint of Taylor & Francis Group, LLC

ISBN: 978-1-032-75374-4 (hbk)
ISBN: 978-1-032-74963-1 (pbk)
ISBN: 978-1-003-47370-1 (ebk)

DOI: 10.1201/9781003473701

Typeset in Palatino
by SPi Technologies India Pvt Ltd (Straive)

Contents

Part III   Vascular Anomalies

Part IV   General

Preface

Anyone who has been a pediatric resident or a pediatric hematology-oncology fellow will remember the anxiety of a night on call. In addition to the relatively common patient with chemotherapy-related fever and neutropenia, there is the anticipation of problems you may have read about but may not have actually seen: the adolescent newly presenting with a white blood cell count of 600,000/mm^3, the 2-year-old spitting up blood with a platelet count of 2,000/mm^3 and a hemoglobin of 5 g/dL, the child who comes to the ER with difficulty walking and is found to have a paraspinal mass on magnetic resonance imaging.

Most issues can wait until the next day when more senior practitioners are around, but some are true medical emergencies and just can't. The tempo with which one needs to come up with a plan for evaluation and treatment will vary—if the service is not too busy, you may have time to pick up a textbook, look at UpToDate or do a PubMed search. Other times, there may be another dozen sick kids on the floor who also need your attention, and your time is more limited.

Our contributors come from a range of generations, but all remember that new-admission anxiety the same way. Apart from guzzling more caffeine before looking for the right information or awakening your attending, we all remember thinking that it might have been nice to have had a quick resource to go to to bridge the hours between the start of night call and morning rounds. There are other housestaff manuals such as the wonderful Harriet Lane *Handbook*, and spiral manuals that give overviews of pathogenesis, diagnostic evaluations and long-term treatment, but none that we know of focuses on what needs to be done immediately to avoid hurting a patient (much less, to avoid looking like a dummy the next day). We offer guidelines to get you started. None is written in stone and some may require institution-based modifications.

We want to thank past University of North Carolina PHO fellows whose Survivors Manual we used in constructing this manual. We also look back gratefully at Dr Richard Sills' model of disease evaluations (*Practical Algorithms in Pediatric Hematology and Oncology*, S. Karger, 2003) that remains very useful. However, we thought that an update was in order, since his edition published in 2003, and that brief step-by-step suggestions focusing on inpatient emergencies could be a big help. To that end, we have compiled 1- to 2-page bullets and algorithms for more than 30 acute emergencies we remember as being the most likely to cause GI distress and sleeplessness. Feel free to suggest other topics or changes that we can make down the line. For those of you who hate algorithms and think that they diminish the thought process a doctor needs to cultivate, we don't disagree—except when it comes to what the first-year fellow or resident must do when alone on call.

You may hate our approach more when you note that we compare the steps we came up with to instructions generated by ChatGPT! For some entries, we have changed the order of bullets to better parallel our own sections; however, the content is faithful to ChatGPT. Spoiler alert: For now, AI just isn't detailed enough, seems geared to the patient rather than the provider, and may already be outdated—although admittedly it does better if you ask it detailed questions. AI may be a better fit in the future, so keep an open mind. We have added a few references for the learner in all of us to go to after some sleep. None of this gets around the need to read definitive texts when time is more flexible!

Acknowledgments

Many thanks to Jonathan Nunez, Senior Director Cybersecurity Researcher & Advisor, for helping us navigate AI terrain; to our fellows, former fellows, and faculty who read through this and gently urged corrections and modifications: Christina Abrams MD (MUSC), A. McCauley Massie MD (UNC), and Kate Westmoreland MD (UNC).

Contributors

Jacquelyn L. Baskin-Miller MD
Division of Pediatric
   Hematology-Oncology
The University of North Carolina
Chapel Hill, North Carolina

Maria O. Boucher MD
Division of Pediatric
   Hematology-Oncology
The University of North Carolina
Chapel Hill, North Carolina

Bridget F. Condit FNP
Division of Pediatric
   Hematology-Oncology
The University of North Carolina
Chapel Hill, North Carolina

Catherine H. Habashy MD MPH
Divisions of Pediatric Hematology-
   Oncology and Hospice and
   Palliative Care
The University of North Carolina
Chapel Hill, North Carolina

Jenna B. Kaplan PharmD
Department of Pharmacy
The University of North Carolina
Chapel Hill, North Carolina

Gerardo Quezada MD
Division of Pediatric
   Hematology-Oncology
The University of North Carolina
Chapel Hill, North Carolina

Abbreviations

ACS	Acute Chest Syndrome
AHTR	Acute Hemolytic Transfusion Reaction
AIHA	Autoimmune Hemolytic Anemia
ALL	Acute Lymphocytic Leukemia
AML	Acute Myelogenous Leukemia
ANC	Absolute Neutrophil Count
APL(APML)	Acute Promyelocytic Leukemia
ATO	Arsenic Trioxide
ATRA	All-Trans Retinoic Acid
AT3	Anti-Thrombin 3
bid	twice a day
BUN	Blood Urea Nitrogen
Ca	Calcium
CBC	Complete Blood Count
CML	Chronic Myelogenous Leukemia
CMP	Complete Metabolic Panel
CNS	Central Nervous System
COG	Children's Oncology Group
Cr	Creatinine
CT	Computed Tomography
CXR	Chest Radiograph
DAT	Direct Antibody Test
DDAVP	Desmopressin Acetate
DIC	Disseminated Intravascular Coagulation
DOAC	Direct Oral Anticoagulant
DVT	Deep Venous Thrombosis
EKG	Electrocardiogram
ER	Emergency Room
FFP	Fresh Frozen Plasma
FH	Fractionated Heparin
FNHTR	Febrile Non-Hemolytic Transfusion Reaction
G6PD	Glucose-6-Phosphate Dehydrogenase
GCSF	Granulocyte Colony Stimulating Factor
GI	Gastrointestine
GVHD	Graft Versus Host Disease
Hgb	Hemoglobin
HIT	Heparin Induced Thrombocytopenia
HLH	Hemophagocytic Lymphohistiocytosis
HS	Hereditary Spherocytosis
(a)HUS	(atypical) Hemolytic Uremic Syndrome
IM	Intramuscular

INR	International Normalized Ratio
I/O	Input/Output
IR	Interventional Radiology
IV	Intravenous
IVC	Inferior Vena Cava
K	Potassium
KMP	Kasabach–Merritt Phenomenon
KVO	Keep Vein Open
LDH	Lactic Dehydrogenase
LFT	Liver Function Tests
LIC	Local Intralesional Clotting
LMWH	Low Molecular Weight Heparin
MAS	Macrophage Activating Syndrome
MCT	Medium-Chain Triglycerides
MCV	Mean Corpuscular Volume
Mg	Magnesium
MISC	Multisystem Inflammatory Syndrome in Children
MPV	Mean Platelet Volume
MRI	Magnetic Resonance Imaging
NHL	Non-Hodgkin Lymphoma
NPO	Nil Per Os (Nothing by Mouth)
NS	Normal Saline
NSAID	Non-Steroidal Anti-Inflammatory Drug
P	Phosphorus
PA	Posterior-Anterior
Pb	Lead
PCA	Patient-Controlled Analgesia
PCR	Polymerase Chain Reaction
PE	Pulmonary Embolus
PFA	Platelet Function Assay
PHO	Pediatric Hematology Oncology
PICU	Pediatric Intensive Care Unit
PIV	Peripheral IV
PIVKA	Proteins Induced by Vitamin K
Plt	Platelet
PRBC	Peripheral Red Blood Cell
PRES	Posterior Reversible Encephalopathy Syndrome
PT	Prothrombin Time
PTT	Partial Thromboplastin Time
PVL	Peripheral Vascular Labs
RAS	Retinoic Acid Syndrome
SCD	Sickle Cell Disease
SL	Sublingual
SVC	Superior Vena Cava
TACO	Transfusion Associated Circulatory Overload
TAR	Thrombocytopenia Absent Radii
tid	three times a day
TLS	Tumor Lysis Syndrome
TMA	Thrombotic MicroAngiopathy

TPA	Tissue Plasminogen Activator
TRALI	Transfusion-Related Acute Lung Injury
TTP	Thrombotic Thrombocytopenic Purpura
UFH	UnFractionated Heparin
UTI	Urinary Tract Infection
VIR	Vascular Interventional Radiology
VM	Vascular Malformation
VOC	Vaso-Occlusive Crisis
VS	Vital Signs
UFH	Unfractionated Heparin
VA	Vascular Anomaly
VM	Vascular Malformation
VWD	Von Willebrand Disease
WBC	White Blood Cell

Note

Italics in text indicate that there is a separate chapter on this topic; **bold** in text indicates emphasis.

Part I

Oncology

1

High White Blood Cell (WBC) Count

Most patients with high WBC, or hyperleukocytosis, will be seen as outpatients. Middle-of-the night admissions for high WBC usually are those suspected of having leukemia. Even most patients with leukemia are not in danger of dying overnight from a high WBC unless it is very high: >200,00/mm^3 at least for patients with acute myeloid leukemia (AML) and arguably >400,000 or 600,000/mm^3 for patients with ALL, and when mostly blasts. The risks are from **hyperviscosity or leukostasis** that can lead to sludging with thrombosis and/or bleeding (notably in the CNS, lung, GI tract), often compounded by other abnormal hematologic parameters (high or low Hgb or platelet levels), concomitant *tumor lysis syndrome with metabolic abnormalities*, or *mediastinal masses*.* We include patients with chronic myelogenous leukemia (CML) in blast crisis. Patients with CML and high WBC in chronic phase and neonates with transient myeloproliferative disorder (*Neonatal Hematologic Emergencies*) do not share this urgency. So, when a patient comes in at 2am **and** after you are sure the patient doesn't need the PICU **and** have assurance from the ER that IV access is adequate (poor IV access may be a reason to send to the PICU):

- Review entire CBC and differential—ideally look at peripheral smear, ordered stat, although this may take an hour or two for the laboratory to have this ready. Is this leukemia and if so, what type is likely?
  - The same sample can be used overnight or the next day for flow cytometry if leukemia is still a concern.
- Order serum chemistries (CMP) stat, including electrolytes, BUN, Cr, LFTs, uric acid, Ca, P, and LDH.
- Type & cross (ask for **irradiated blood products** unless you are sure this isn't malignancy): Don't transfuse (somewhat arbitrarily) above Hgb 8g/dL to minimize worsening any hyperviscosity.
- Start hydration with D5 ½NS even before other labs are available (there is not a downside if this turns out not to be leukemia)—1–2× maintenance and **no K (Ringer's Lactate has a small amount of K and we recommend avoiding it)**. No need for alkalinization. Hyperleukocytosis can cause **pseudohyperkalemia** (check K on blood gas and get EKG to look for T waves if you are unsure); too little K is better than too much.

---

* *Italics* in text indicate that there is a separate chapter on this topic; **bold** in text indicates emphasis.

DOI: 10.1201/9781003473701-2

- If elevated uric acid: see *Tumor Lysis Syndrome*
- If elevated P, low Ca, etc.: *Tumor Lysis Syndrome*
- Start allopurinol 10 mg/kg/day divided tid PO, or rasburicase (at our institution: <30 kg: 1.5 mg IV once, >30 kg: 3 mg IV once for ALL with WBC ≥ 100,000/mm^3 or AML with WBC ≥50,000/mm^3 if uric acid is ≥8 mg/dL and for all other oncology patients if uric acid is ≥12 mg/dL, where 9 mg/dL is upper limit of normal). There may be institutional restrictions on rasburicase so check with your pharmacy. You can order for 4 more days or wait until the morning—one dose is typically enough and you often can revert to allopurinol. **Check G6PD** for patients at high risk of deficiency (i.e., African-American males or those of Middle-Eastern background) **before** rasburicase.
- Keep platelet count >10,000/mm^3 (>50,000/mm^3 if procedures anticipated).
- History including recent systemic corticosteroid use, **menstrual status and expected next period** (to be sure bleeding is not imminent).
- Physical examination including vital signs (VS) with height and weight (to allow dose calculations), look for adenopathy, liver and spleen size, neurologic status, and do not forget genital exam especially in males to be sure that there is no age-inappropriate enlargement or mass to suggest testicular involvement.
- Talk with the patient and family to tell them the plan!
- Be sure that the patient is metabolically stable (normal K, Cr, uric acid) before starting cytotoxics including hydroxyurea (hydrea) or steroids. **Try to avoid steroids** overnight—they may interfere with subsequent protocol eligibility (some would say don't use at all without talking with your attending). The use of hydroxyurea in patients with CML is arguable. A short course may be given in symptomatic patients with high leukocyte or platelet counts while molecular and cytogenetic confirmation of the CML diagnosis is pending. Doses are age as well as size dependent so look it up if you start with a few days of hydrea.
- CXR (ideally done on the way up for admission from the ER): this should be a posterior–anterior (PA) and lateral film if possible.
- Consider calling transfusion medicine on-call if the standard of practice is for leukapheresis—this likely won't happen for hours except as a "push-pull" through a peripheral IV and by that time the WBC may have come down considerably from hydration alone. Leukapheresis usually requires a PICU stay and is only a temporary measure until chemotherapy can be started.
- Make NPO (nothing by mouth) in case procedures will be needed in the AM.
- Monitor I/O, repeat chemistries every 6 hours initially (and remember to check results).
- Consider calling on-call Nephrology if concerns about need for dialysis.
- If you are a Children's Oncology Group (or other consortium) member, take a look at relevant COG (or other group) protocols and look at "Requirements": https://childrensoncologygroup.org/.
- We think these patients do best on a pediatric oncology floor but this may vary with institution, and a PICU may be the better venue for patients with very high WBC at some centers.

Bibliography

Aylan Gelen S, Sarper N, Zengin E, Azizoğlu MJ. Management of Hyperleukocytosis in Childhood Acute Leukemia without Leukapheresis and Rasburicase Prophylaxis. *Pediatr Hematol Oncol.* 2022;44:12–18.

Golubella A, Thooft A, Antoine P, et al. Pseudo-hyperkalemia and Hyperleukocytosis. *Rev Med Brux.* 2013;34:179–180.

Leung KKY, Hon KL, Hui WF, et al. Therapeutics for Paediatric Oncological emergencies. *Drugs Context.* 2021;10:1–12.

What ChatGPT Says

Pretty vague and not much detail for that first night admission

1. *Diagnosis*:
   a. Medical history and physical examination.
   b. *Complete blood count (CBC)*: CBC … Hyperleukocytosis is typically defined as a white blood cell count greater than 100,000 cells per microliter (µL) of blood.
   c. Peripheral blood smear.
   d. *Bone marrow aspiration and biopsy*: A bone marrow examination may be necessary to determine the cause of hyperleukocytosis, especially if leukemia is suspected.
   e. *Additional tests*: … flow cytometry, cytogenetic analysis, and molecular genetic testing.
2. *Management*: The management of hyperleukocytosis depends on the underlying cause and the patient's clinical condition. Here are some general principles:
3. *Supportive care*: Patients with hyperleukocytosis may require supportive care to manage symptoms, such as fever, infection, and bleeding. This may include antibiotics, transfusions of blood products (e.g., platelets or red blood cells), and medications to control symptoms.
4. *Treatment of underlying cause*:
   a. *Leukemia*: If hyperleukocytosis is due to leukemia, treatment typically involves chemotherapy and sometimes radiation therapy or stem cell transplantation.
   b. *Infection or Inflammation*: Address the underlying infection or inflammatory condition with appropriate medications and treatments.
5. *Leukapheresis*: In cases of extreme hyperleukocytosis with a high risk of complications (e.g., severe respiratory distress or neurological symptoms), leukapheresis may be considered. … This is typically a short-term measure to stabilize the patient's condition.
6. *Monitoring*: Continuous monitoring of the patient's clinical status, blood counts, and response to treatment is essential.

Algorithm: **High White Blood Cell (WBC) Count**

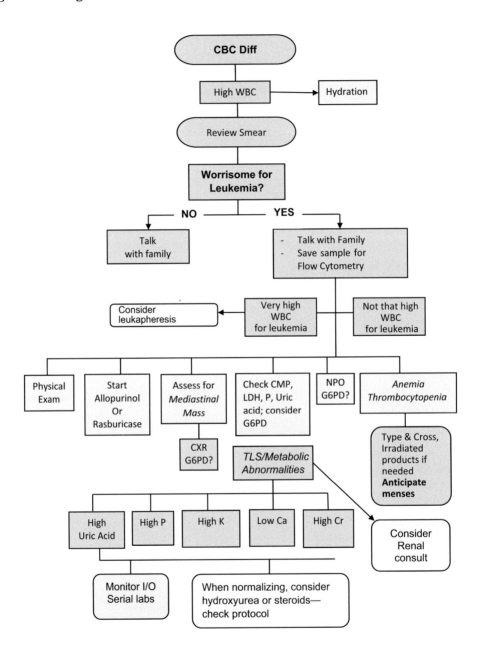

2

Mediastinal Mass/Superior Vena Cava (SVC) Syndrome

Mediastinal masses can involve the posterior, mid, or anterior mediastinum. Typically, it is the anterior mediastinal masses that are middle-of-the-night issues. The terrible "4 T's of the anterior mediastinum" are teratomas, thyroid masses, thymomas, and most commonly T-cell lymphomas. Middle mediastinal masses also can cause issues. Non-Hodgkin lymphomas (NHL) are the most likely to cause SVC syndrome, which is characterized by variable degrees of facial swelling, plethora, orthopnea, coughing, hoarseness, venous distension of the neck. SVC syndrome is uncommon with Hodgkin's disease, since most of these in pediatrics are nodular sclerosis and the fibrosis (sclerosis) keeps the mass from collapsing on the trachea. Mediastinal masses due to T-cell ALL or NHL commonly are seen in adolescent males and often occur together with *high WBC counts* and metabolic abnormalities of leukemia including hyperkalemia, hyperuricemia, hyper- or hypocalcemia, hyperphosphatemia, and renal failure (*TLS/Metabolic Abnormalities*). The major emergency faced by these patients specifically from the mass is respiratory failure due to tracheal compression. This can be sudden, life-threatening, and is compounded by sedation of any sort not just general anesthesia. Until you have a diagnosis and when the diagnosis is leukemia-lymphoma or just lymphoma, do the following:

- Review a posterior–anterior (PA) and lateral chest X-ray (CXR) to look for airway (tracheal or bronchial) compression, which can be seen on plain films. The larger the mass the more likely there will be problems. In the world of lymphomas, bulk disease is defined as a mass diameter >1/3 the diameter of the chest, with the latter measured at the level of the diaphragm;

- If a bone marrow aspirate is planned urgently (and that is rarely needed overnight), **do not sedate** the patient without anesthesia clearance—marrows can be done with the patient sitting up, and local numbing medicine;

- Physical examination including vital signs with height and weight (to allow dose calculations), look for plethora, venous distension in the neck, adenopathy that might offer a peripheral site to biopsy if the bone marrow is non-diagnostic, liver-spleen size, neurologic status, Tanner staging and be sure that there is no age-inappropriate enlargement or mass to suggest testicular involvement;

- Keep the patient's head elevated and have the patient remain supine;

- If major tracheal compression on CXR, patient may do better in the PICU for monitoring;

- Call for an anesthesia consult. If there is tracheal obstruction, tracheostomy may not help if the obstruction is below trach placement. Anesthesia may have to force

DOI: 10.1201/9781003473701-3

an intratracheal tube past the obstruction—not always easy and an experienced anesthesiologist will need to be around;

- Sometimes treatment is needed to relieve tracheal compression before a biopsy can be done safely—methylprednisolone 20 mg/m^2 IV tid is one possibility (after you are sure that the patient is metabolically normal), with ongoing monitoring for tumor lysis.

Bibliography

Hastings CA, Torkildson JC, Agrawal AK, eds. *Handbook of Pediatric Hematology and Oncology: Children's Hospital & Research Center Oakland*. 2nd edition. John Wiley & Sons Ltd. 2012.

Leung KKY, Hon KL, Hui WF, et al. Therapeutics for paediatric oncological emergencies. *Drugs Context*. 2021;10:2020-11-5.

What ChatGTP Says

We asked ChatGPT about each of these terms separately. The overviews are not bad, but they are vague and do not provide nuanced help for night-call cover. It does give a differential diagnosis for SVC syndrome, whereas we focus in this section on mediastinal masses as a reason for SVC syndrome.

Mediastinal Mass

1. Medical history and physical examination

2. *Imaging studies*: Imaging is crucial for locating and characterizing the mediastinal mass. Common imaging tests include:

   a. Chest X-ray: A chest X-ray may be the initial screening test and can provide an overview of the mass's location and size.

   b. *Computed Tomography (CT) scan*: A CT scan provides detailed images of the mediastinum, allowing for better localization, characterization, and assessment of the mass's relationship to nearby structures.

   c. *Magnetic Resonance Imaging (MRI)*: An MRI may be used when additional detail is needed, particularly in evaluating soft tissue structures within the mediastinum.

   d. *Positron emission tomography (PET) scan*: A PET scan can help determine if the mass is metabolically active and whether it might be cancerous.

3. *Biopsy*: In most cases, a biopsy is necessary to determine the nature of the mass. This can be done through various methods:

   a. Fine-needle aspiration (FNA…

   b. Core biopsy…

   c. *Surgical biopsy*: In some cases, a surgical procedure (mediastinoscopy, thoracoscopy, or thoracotomy) may be necessary to obtain a tissue sample.

    d. *Laboratory tests*: Blood tests may be performed to assess the patient's general health and check for tumor markers or other specific markers associated with certain conditions.

4. *Management*: Management of a mediastinal mass depends on its underlying cause, which can vary widely. Treatment options may include:

    a. *Observation*: In some cases, particularly when the mass is small, non-specific, and not causing symptoms, close observation (watchful waiting) …

    b. *Surgical removal*: … The extent and complexity of the surgery will depend on the location and nature of the mass.

    c. *Radiation therapy*: Radiation therapy may be used in combination with surgery or as a primary treatment for certain types of mediastinal masses, such as thymomas.

    d. *Chemotherapy*: Chemotherapy is used to treat certain mediastinal masses, particularly those that are malignant or have metastasized to other parts of the body.

    e. *Targeted therapy and immunotherapy*: These approaches may be considered for specific types of mediastinal masses, especially if they have specific molecular or genetic features.

    f. Follow-up…

SVC Syndrome

Superior vena cava (SVC) syndrome is a medical emergency that occurs when there is partial or complete obstruction of the superior vena cava… It can result from various causes, such as tumors, blood clots, or inflammation.

1. *Diagnosis*:

    a. *Clinical assessment*: SVC syndrome typically presents with symptoms that can include swelling of the face, neck, and upper chest, as well as difficulty breathing, coughing, and visible veins on the chest and neck.

    b. *Imaging studies*: (overlap with Mediastinal Mass, so here are some additional points): computed tomography (CT) scan or magnetic resonance imaging (MRI): These tests provide detailed images of the chest, allowing for the localization and characterization of the obstruction and the identification of any underlying masses or blood clots.

       • *Venography*: In some cases, a venogram may be performed to visualize the blocked blood flow in the superior vena cava.

2. *Management*:

    a. *Immediate stabilization*: If the patient has severe symptoms or is in respiratory distress, the immediate goal is to stabilize the patient. This may include providing oxygen, elevating the head of the bed, and offering medications to relieve symptoms.

    b. *Treating the underlying cause*:

       • *Tumor-related SVC syndrome*: If a tumor is identified as the cause, treatment may involve chemotherapy, radiation therapy, or surgery to shrink or remove the tumor. In some cases, a stent may be placed to keep the vein open.

- *Thrombotic SVC syndrome*: If the obstruction is due to a blood clot, anticoagulant medications (blood thinners) may be prescribed to dissolve the clot.

c. *Symptom management*: Medications and interventions may be used to manage symptoms such as pain, swelling, and difficulty breathing.

d. *Endovascular stent placement*: In some cases, a vascular surgeon may insert a stent into the superior vena cava to keep it open and restore blood flow. This procedure can provide rapid relief of symptoms.

e. *Supportive care*: Patients with SVC syndrome may require supportive care to manage complications such as infection or clot formation.

f. Close monitoring.

Algorithm: **Mediastinal Mass/Superior Vena Cava (SVC) Syndrome**

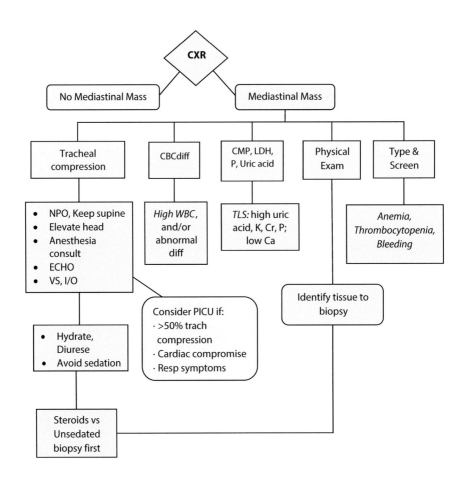

3

Spinal/Paraspinal Mass

Spinal/paraspinal mass can present as emergency diagnostic or therapeutic dilemmas. The differential diagnosis is broad and ranges from benign and malignant tumors, infections such as tuberculosis, to hematomas from coagulopathies or trauma (the latter don't usually come to PHO). Suspicion is the start of good management. Tempo is critical since paraplegias become irreversible or at least hard to reverse over time (some say >48 hours). For patients with known malignancy but before imaging has been done, new back pain should be assumed to be due to epidural compression until proven otherwise. For all patients, including those in whom the reason for pain is less certain, evaluation may begin before transfer to PHO but should include:

- History: The presentation will depend on location but may include pain over at least one part of the spine, paresthesias, weakness in lower extremities for thoraco-lumbar masses or in the upper extremities for C-spine or high thoracic lesions, and bowel-bladder symptoms. In some cases, imaging will be the first indication of a mass;
  - Establish context (does the patient have *hemophilia*, low platelets, known cancer or systemic signs that suggest a new cancer diagnosis such as fever, weight loss; history of easy bleeding even without a specific diagnosis; was there a history of trauma?);
- Physical examination should be complete but with a more detailed neuro exam than usual to document weakness—tone, strength, reflexes, and sensory level will serve both as a baseline and a reason for imaging studies. Even at night, you can call a neurology consultant who presumably will do a better neuro exam than you!
- Imaging: Confirmation is critical and imaging may well have been done in the ER before transfer to the floor. If not, and if suspicion is high enough, an urgent MRI with and without contrast is the gold standard. Plain radiographs of the spine and an uncontrasted CT scan (faster and more realistic to get overnight) are indicated if you can't get an MRI emergently;
- Talk to the patient and family and tell them what you are thinking/planning. Not a bad idea at this point to call your attending who will not be happy if he/she/they arrives in the morning and finds a paretic patient without having been forewarned;

DOI: 10.1201/9781003473701-4

- While you are waiting (and waiting and waiting and calling radiology to remind them of the urgency), draw bloodwork: CBC diff, chem screen with LDH and uric acid if cancer is on the list, coags (PT/INR, PTT and ask about bleeding history) and a type & cross in case surgery is needed;
- Although corticosteroids (dexamethasone in Harriet Lane Handbook dosing for spinal cord compression is reasonable) can help acutely with edema, **don't start until you are sure that the patient is metabolically normal**—lymphomatous masses can cause cord compression and *tumor lysis syndrome* can be an issue that should be addressed before starting steroids;
- Definitive treatment will depend on the diagnosis (surgery, antibiotics, chemo-therapy, radiation therapy). However, if symptoms are severe or progressive, "generic" treatment may need to precede diagnosis:
  - Once a mass is documented, consider calling radiation oncology and neurosur-gery to give them a heads-up. Surgery has the advantage of providing tissue if diagnosis is uncertain but laminectomy may have more long-term conse-quences than radiation. You can let radiation oncology and neurosurgery duke it out, but we usually try to avoid laminectomy. Chemotherapy with cyclophos-phamide may be a good option for malignancy even before a tissue diagnosis (see *Mediastinal Mass, Massive Hepatomegaly*);
- Go easy on pain meds to allow monitoring of signs and symptoms.

Bibliography

Rheingold SR, Li AM, Freedman JL. Medical emergencies. In Blaney SM, Adamson PC, Helman L, eds, *Pizzo & Poplack's Pediatric Oncology*, 8th ed., Wolters Kluwer, 2021: Ch 34.

What ChatGPT Says

Not bad as an overview, but short on details.

These masses can arise from various sources, including tumors, infections, cysts, or other structural abnormalities. Here is a general outline of the diagnostic and management steps:

1. *Diagnosis*:
   a. *Clinical assessment*: A thorough medical history and physical examination… Symptoms may include back pain, neurological deficits, weakness, or sensory changes.

b. *Imaging studies*: Diagnostic imaging is crucial for localizing and characterizing the spinal or paraspinal mass. Common imaging tests include:

- X-rays: Initial screening to visualize bone structures and any gross abnormalities.
- Computed tomography (CT) scan: Provides detailed cross-sectional images to assess the mass, its size, and its relationship to surrounding structures.
- Magnetic resonance imaging (MRI): Offers high-resolution images to evaluate soft tissues and assess the extent of the mass and its impact on the spinal cord and nerves.
- Positron emission tomography (PET) scan: May be used to determine whether the mass is metabolically active, which can be important in diagnosing cancerous lesions.

c. *Biopsy*: To determine the nature of the mass and whether it is benign or malignant, a biopsy may be required. Biopsies can be performed percutaneously (using a needle through the skin), surgically, or during spinal surgery, depending on the location and nature of the mass.

d. *Laboratory tests*: Blood tests may be conducted to evaluate the general health of the patient and to check for markers that could be associated with certain conditions, such as infection or cancer.

2. *Management*:

The management of a spinal or paraspinal mass depends on its underlying cause and whether it is causing symptoms or neurological deficits. Treatment options may include:

a. *Observation*: In some cases, particularly when the mass is small, non-specific, and not causing symptoms, a "watch and wait" approach may be recommended to monitor any changes over time.

b. *Surgical removal*: If the mass is causing neurological deficits or is likely to be cancerous, surgical removal may be necessary. The extent of surgery and approach depends on the location and nature of the mass.

c. *Radiation therapy*: Radiation therapy may be used in combination with surgery or as a primary treatment for certain spinal or paraspinal masses, especially those that are malignant or inoperable.

d. *Chemotherapy*: Chemotherapy is used to treat certain types of cancerous spinal or paraspinal masses, particularly if they have metastasized to other parts of the body.

e. *Steroid treatment*: Corticosteroids may be used to reduce inflammation and swelling, particularly when the mass is compressing the spinal cord and causing neurological deficits.

f. *Supportive care*: Patients may require supportive care to manage pain, neurological symptoms, and complications.

Algorithm: **Spinal/Paraspinal Mass**

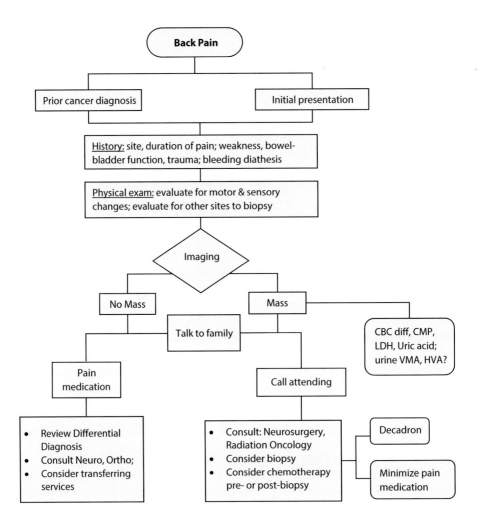

4

Massive Hepatomegaly

Very large livers, those palpated or reported on radiographic studies to extend to the level of the umbilicus and even to the pelvic brim, are most commonly seen by pediatric hematology oncology in the newborn period. Although there are non-oncologic reasons for massive hepatomegaly (e.g., glycogen storage diseases), in neonates and infants under 18 months of age, massive livers are most commonly due to neuroblastoma. In older patients, CML may need to be considered (see *High WBC Count*). The good news is that neuroblastoma in infants usually is what is referred to as **International Neuroblastoma Staging System (INSS) 4S**—"special" stage 4—characterized by a small primary tumor often in an adrenal gland and metastatic disease usually limited to the skin, bone marrow, and liver. The overall outcome of infants with stage 4S neuroblastoma is excellent and ≥80% are cured. In some cases, the tumor resolves on its own over time. The bad news is that a cure, even if that is the ultimate result, doesn't always come easily. Middle-of-the-night emergencies that the on-call person may need to evaluate usually are due to mass effect from the liver: renal failure from extrinsic compression of the kidneys, gut necrosis from intestinal obstruction, and especially respiratory embarrassment from upward displacement of the diaphragm. Liver failure and coagulopathy may be emergency issues as well. Some patients may be seen after another service has obtained imaging that identifies a primary adrenal or *paraspinal mass* strongly suggesting the diagnosis. Even if that is not the case, think about these overnight steps:

- This is one case where a good physical examination should come first: In addition to documenting the size of the liver, obtain vital signs to look for: respiratory failure (respiratory rate and pulse, blood pressure, oxygen saturation; weight to help with monitoring Is/Os and drug dosing, and abdominal girth); Are breath sounds diminished or is the baby having intercostal retractions? Examine the skin to look for blueberry muffin lesions, which are not pathognomonic but will point to a diagnosis of neuroblastoma and will give you something to have biopsied the next day. Is there edema or reduced pulses in the legs from tumor compression?
- History: fevers, icterus, bruising, weight gain or loss, travel or transfusion exposures, family history of storage disorders;
- Talk with the family to tell them the plan;
- Continuous monitoring of O_2 saturation and VS including weights and abdominal girth will be helpful;
- Consider a Foley catheter to monitor Is and Os;

DOI: 10.1201/9781003473701-5

- As with other settings suggestive of cancer: blood draw for CBC and differential, serum chemistries stat including electrolytes, BUN, Cr, LFTs, uric acid, Ca, P, LDH, Type & cross (ask for irradiated blood products unless you are sure this isn't malignancy, see *Transfusion Emergencies*) and INR, PTT if you can get enough blood;
- Urine for random levels of vanillylmandelic acid (VMA) and homovanillic acid (HVA) even though this will take a few days to result;
- Start hydration with D5 ½ NS or NS even before other labs are available—1× maintenance may be fine and **no K (Ringer's lactate has a small amount of K, and we recommend avoiding it)**. If uric acid is elevated or electrolytes are abnormal, see *TLS/Metabolic Abnormalities*;
- Good IV access for imaging, serial blood draws, and supportive care—this may require PICU;
- Overnight, observation usually is enough intervention and you can talk about diagnostic studies in the morning. If organ failure is imminent, options (which will require discussion before implementing, since diagnosis may be suspected but not yet certain) include:
  - Cytotoxic chemotherapy—one regimen from an old COG protocol starts with carboplatin 560 mg/m^2 or 18 mg/kg IV over 1 hour, and etoposide 120 mg/m^2 or 4 mg/kg IV over 2 hours. Another easier regimen is cyclophosphamide 5 mg/kg/day IV over 1 hour daily for 5 days, both with IV fluids. Ongoing chemo and possible use of G-CSF can be discussed in the AM;
  - Hepatic artery chemo-embolization which is not clearly more effective or less toxic than IV chemo and requires buy-in from interventional radiology;
  - Low-dose radiation therapy usually can't be started on nights and most people don't use it for this indication.

Bibliography

Weintraub M, Waldman E, Koplewitz B, et al. A sequential treatment algorithm for infants with stage 4s neuroblastoma and massive hepatomegaly. *Pediatr Blood Cancer*. 2012;5:182–184.

What ChatGPT Says

Pretty vague and not much help with regard to emergency measures. Treatment guidelines don't take cancer into account:

1. *Diagnosis*:
   a. *Clinical assessment*: A comprehensive medical history and a thorough physical examination... inquire about any recent illnesses, medications, dietary habits, family history, and exposure to toxins.
   b. *Imaging studies*:
      - Abdominal ultrasound: This is often the first-line imaging study to evaluate the size, shape, and structure of the liver and identify any gross abnormalities.
      - Computed tomography (CT) scan or magnetic resonance imaging (MRI): These tests can provide more detailed images to assess the cause of hepatomegaly and its impact on surrounding structures.
   c. *Blood tests*: liver function tests bilirubin levels, and markers of liver disease. Specific tests may also be performed to check for viral hepatitis, metabolic disorders, autoimmune diseases, or other conditions that can affect the liver.
   d. *Genetic testing*: In cases of suspected metabolic or genetic disorders, genetic testing may be necessary to identify the underlying genetic mutations responsible for the hepatomegaly.
   e. *Biopsy*: A liver biopsy may be required...

2. *Management*:
   The management of massive hepatomegaly in childhood depends on the underlying cause and the child's clinical condition. Treatment options may include:
   a. *Treatment of the underlying cause*:
      - *Viral hepatitis*: If hepatomegaly is caused by viral hepatitis, specific antiviral medications may be prescribed.
      - *Metabolic disorders*: Management may involve dietary modifications, enzyme replacement therapy, or other specific treatments for inborn errors of metabolism.
      - *Autoimmune liver diseases*: Immunosuppressive medications, such as corticosteroids or other immunosuppressants, may be necessary to manage autoimmune liver conditions.
   b. *Management of symptoms*: Treatment may include addressing symptoms such as abdominal pain, jaundice, or pruritus with medications or lifestyle modifications.

Algorithm: **Massive Hepatomegaly**

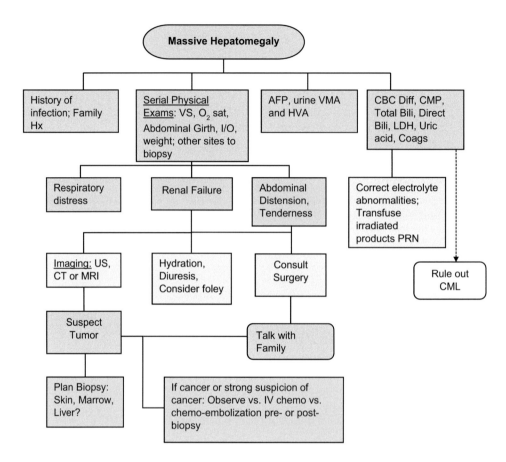

5

Tumor Lysis Syndrome (TLS)/Metabolic Abnormalities

Tumor lysis syndrome (TLS) with metabolic abnormalities can occur with either spontaneous or chemotherapy-induced cancer cell lysis. It is most likely to arise in the setting of leukemia or NHL (especially Burkitt lymphoma) or other cancers with rapidly dividing cells, and manifests as hyperkalemia, hyperphosphatemia with secondary hypocalcemia, and hyperuricemia. These metabolic abnormalities can cause renal failure, arrhythmias, seizures, and even death. Although TLS can be present at diagnosis, the greatest risk of TLS is 12–72 hours after starting chemotherapy. An ounce of prevention includes:

- Hydration with 1.5–2x maintenance (NO POTASSIUM) or 125 mL/m^2/h ½NS or D5 ½NS. No need for alkalinization. **Ringer's lactate has a small amount of K and we recommend avoiding it**;

- Start allopurinol. When uric acid is very high (maybe >8 mg/dL, and your institution may have guidelines), consider rasburicase (see *High White Blood Cell Count* for doses);

- At least daily weights, and careful I/O which may require placement of a Foley catheter; diuresis with Lasix (maybe 0.5 mg/kg IV, max 20 mg) as needed to get O=I and to keep weight from increasing;

- TLS labs stat q6-8hr at least overnight, depending on initial abnormalities: Basic metabolic panel, P, Ca, Uric Acid. Remember, hyperkalemia can be an artifact of red cells or tumor lysis in the blood collection tube. If rasburicase is used, the sample should immediately be **placed on ice** to avoid continued uricase activity and a falsely reassuring low uric acid level;

- Sometimes a pound of cure is needed if TLS is underway. Apart from suspecting TLS, treatment recommendations in addition to the measures listed above address specific metabolic abnormalities:

  - **Hyperkalemia**: obtain EKG and consider EKG monitor looking for peaked T waves. If these are noted proceed with rapid correction, and consider transfer to PICU. Consult the on-call nephrologist as dialysis may be needed. You or PICU may need to correct high K with 50 mg/kg calcium gluconate (max 2 grams), 0.1 unit/kg insulin (max 5 units), 5 mL/kg D10;

  - Lab recheck 60 minutes after intervention; can repeat if necessary. Too low a K is safer than too high. Beware pseudo-hyperkalemia and check a blood gas or whole blood potassium (see *High WBC*);

DOI: 10.1201/9781003473701-6

- **Hyperphosphatemia**: start with aluminum hydroxide (30 mg/kg/dose tid with meals—max 640 mg tid, but avoid if kidney disease is present) or sevelamer (children 400 mg tid with meals, adolescents 800–1,600 mg tid with meals);
- **Hypocalcemia**: Check albumin (**low albumin will make the free Ca look low**). **Correct hyperphosphatemia** to avoid deposition of calcium phosphate salts when IV calcium is given. Check Mg and **correct hypomagnesemia**, which impairs parathyroid hormone (PTH) response and correction of low calcium. If symptomatic, treat with IV calcium chloride or calcium gluconate. Anticipate bradycardia and consider PICU.

Bibliography

Leung KKY, Hon KL, Hui WF, et al. Therapeutics for Paediatric Oncological Emergencies. *Drugs Context*. 2021;10:1–12.

What ChatGPT Says

More or less the same talking points, and a good overview, but not enough detail.

Tumor lysis syndrome (TLS) is a potentially life-threatening medical emergency that can occur in individuals with cancer, typically after the initiation of cancer treatment. TLS is characterized by the rapid release of intracellular contents, such as potassium, phosphorus, and nucleic acids, into the bloodstream as cancer cells are destroyed. The resulting metabolic imbalances can lead to complications, including kidney dysfunction, cardiac arrhythmias, seizures, and even death. Prompt diagnosis and management are essential. Here are the key steps in the diagnosis and management of tumor lysis syndrome:

1. *Diagnosis*:
   a. *Clinical assessment*: … be vigilant for TLS in patients at risk, which includes those with high tumor burden, certain types of cancer (e.g., high-grade lymphomas, acute leukemias), and those initiating cancer treatment.
   b. *Laboratory tests*:
      - *Electrolyte levels*: Frequent monitoring of potassium, phosphorus, calcium, and uric acid levels is essential. Elevated levels of these electrolytes are indicative of TLS.

- *Kidney function*: Blood urea nitrogen (BUN) and serum creatinine levels should be monitored to assess kidney function. An increase in these values may suggest renal impairment.
- *Urinalysis*: Urinalysis may reveal uric acid crystals, hematuria (blood in urine), or signs of kidney damage.

c. *EKG (Electrocardiogram)*: An EKG may be performed to assess cardiac function and detect any abnormalities, such as arrhythmias, which can occur as a result of electrolyte imbalances.

2. *Management*:

Management of TLS involves a combination of preventive measures and treatments aimed at correcting metabolic imbalances, protecting kidney function, and managing complications. The specific approach may vary depending on the severity of TLS.

a. *Hydration*: Adequate hydration is crucial to maintain urine flow and help flush out excess electrolytes and metabolic byproducts. Intravenous (IV) fluids, typically isotonic saline, should be administered to maintain urine output.

b. *Allopurinol or rasburicase*: These medications are used to lower uric acid levels and prevent uric acid crystallization. Rasburicase is more effective in rapidly reducing uric acid levels and is often preferred in severe cases.

c. *Phosphate binders*: These can be administered to lower elevated phosphate levels in the blood.

d. *Calcium gluconate*: In severe hyperkalemia (high blood potassium levels) or as a preventive treatment, calcium gluconate may be administered to stabilize cardiac cell membranes.

e. *Hemodialysis*: In cases of severe kidney dysfunction or life-threatening metabolic abnormalities, hemodialysis may be required to rapidly remove excess electrolytes and waste products from the blood.

f. *Monitor and treat complications*: Prompt treatment of complications such as cardiac arrhythmias, seizures, and acute kidney injury is essential. Symptomatic management may *include* anti-arrhythmics, anticonvulsants, and renal replacement therapy.

g. *Close monitoring*: Regular monitoring of electrolyte levels, kidney function, and overall clinical status is crucial. Adjustments to treatment should be made, based on these assessments.

Prevention of TLS is a key component in managing cancer patients at risk. Strategies include risk assessment, hydration protocols, and prophylactic use of medications like allopurinol or rasburicase. The specific approach to prevention and management should be individualized based on the patient's condition.

Algorithm: Tumor Lysis Syndrome (TLS)/Metabolic Abnormalities

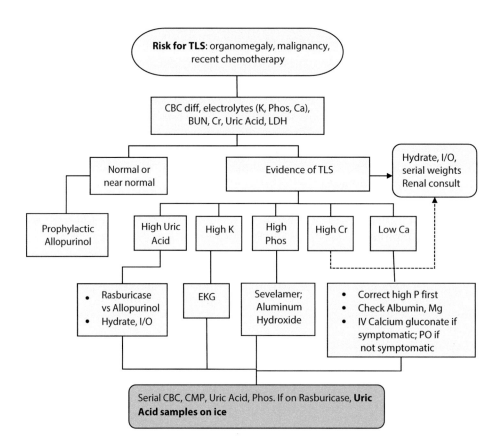

6

Differentiation Syndrome or Retinoic Acid Syndrome

This is characterized by three or more of the following: respiratory distress, hypoxemia, fever, erythematous rash, pulmonary infiltrates, pleural or pericardial effusions, weight gain, peripheral edema, acute renal failure, congestive heart failure, and hypotension. Differentiation Syndrome (DS), also called Retinoic Acid Syndrome (RAS), is seen almost exclusively in the context of a patient with new or relapsed acute promyelocytic leukemia (APL or APML) starting treatment with all-trans retinoic acid (ATRA) and/or arsenic tri-oxide (ATO). It is not reported with cis-retinoic acid as used in solid tumors. Suspicion is 9/10 of treatment. Current Children's Oncology Group (COG) studies have incorporated prophylactic dexamethasone for high-risk APL (WBC $\geq$ 10,000/mm^3) at 2.5 mg/m^2/dose PO or IV, twice daily for 14 days (see COG protocol if you are a member). If DS occurs with or without prophylaxis:

- Stop ATRA and ATO (may be able to restart at a later date but not your problem for tonight);
- Supportive care as needed with O$_2$, furosemide for fluid overload and pressors;
- Start dexamethasone 5.8 mg/m^2/dose IV bid (max 10 mg/dose bid, even for patients already on prophylaxis) for a minimum of 3 days and continue until resolution of symptoms, then continue at a prophylactic dose through day 14;
- Supportive care with O$_2$, IV fluids size of;
- For patients with standard risk APL, if the WBC count rises above 10,000/mm^3, add hydroxyurea;
- Most DS can be managed on a regular medical floor but PICU transfer may be needed;
- Talk with patient and family to let them know the plan;
- Baseline and serial coagulation tests (PT/INR and PTT) are indicated in patients with APL but are not necessarily related to DS. Correct these with treatment of underlying APL, blood products as needed (keep fibrinogen >150 mg/dL, platelets >30,000/mm^3), and avoid invasive procedures.

Bibliography

Stahl M, Tallman MS. Differentiation syndrome in acute promyelocytic leukaemia. *Br J Haematol.* 2019;187:157–162.

What ChatGPT Says

Not bad, though without the detail an on-call person will need.

1. *Diagnosis*:
   a. *Clinical assessment*: Healthcare providers should be vigilant for signs and symptoms of differentiation syndrome in patients with APL undergoing treatment with medications such as all-trans retinoic acid (ATRA) or arsenic trioxide (ATO). Symptoms typically develop within the first 10–20 days of treatment.
   b. *Common symptoms*: … include fever, weight gain, respiratory distress, pleural or pericardial effusions (fluid accumulation in the chest or heart lining), and organ dysfunction, low blood pressure, pulmonary infiltrates, kidney dysfunction, and skin rashes.
   c. *Laboratory tests*:
      • *Blood counts*: Complete blood counts (CBC) should be monitored for any changes in white blood cell, red blood cell, and platelet counts.
      • *Coagulation profile*: Coagulation tests may be performed to assess the risk of bleeding or clotting.
      • *Imaging*: Chest X-rays or CT scans may be done to evaluate for the presence of pleural or pericardial effusions.

2. *Management*:
   Management of differentiation syndrome involves promptly addressing the symptoms and discontinuing or adjusting the ATRA or ATO treatment. The specific approach may vary depending on the severity of the syndrome:
   a. *Discontinue or adjust treatment*: The first step is to halt or reduce the dose of ATRA or ATO to alleviate the differentiation syndrome. Treatment may be resumed once the symptoms have resolved.
   b. *Corticosteroids*: High-dose corticosteroids, such as dexamethasone, are often used to control the inflammatory response and manage symptoms like fever, respiratory distress, and organ dysfunction.
   c. *Supportive care*: Supportive measures, including oxygen therapy and fluid management, may be required to address respiratory distress and organ dysfunction.
   d. *Cardiac evaluation*: If differentiation syndrome causes cardiac symptoms (e.g., pericardial effusion), a cardiologist may need to evaluate and manage the cardiac component.
   e. *Close monitoring*: Frequent monitoring of the patient's clinical status, vital signs, blood counts, and organ function is essential. Adjustments to the treatment plan should be made based on these assessments.

Algorithm: Differentiation Syndrome or Retinoic Acid Syndrome

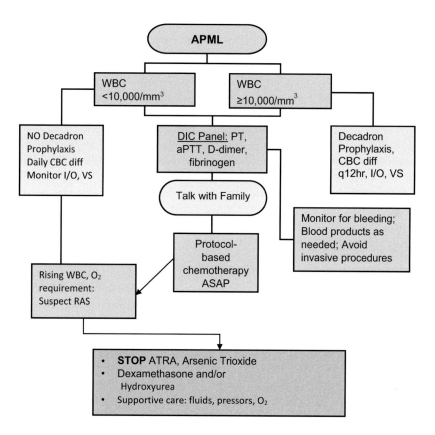

7

Fever in High-Risk Populations

Patients with fever at high risk for serious infection include patients with severe neutropenia (ANC < 500/mm^3) or impending neutropenia (those about to drop their ANC from recent chemotherapy), those with central lines, primary or secondary immunodeficiency syndromes, sickle cell disease (SCD), and others with functional or anatomic asplenia, (including those with polysplenia), or very young babies with vascular malformations. The definition of fever is a bit arbitrary but we **don't** adjust for how temperature is taken (oral, skin, and the usually proscribed rectal temps). One guideline is a temperature of 101°F (38.3°C) once or multiple temperatures of ≥100.4° (38.0°C) in one day or even once in an ill-appearing child. Not all fever is due to infection, but the better part of valor in these high-risk patients is to assume sepsis until proven otherwise. In many cases, most of the evaluation and start of treatment will happen in an ER (although the on-call fellow may be the one to provide guidelines to outside ERs and to decide who needs to be admitted). Apart from ill-appearing patients with any diagnosis (with or without neutropenia) and severely neutropenic patients, most patients with fever can be managed as outpatients. For children with SCD, **consideration of admission** also should be given for those with temperatures >39°C, WBC >30,000/mm^3, or WBC <5,000/mm^3, age <12 months, history of bacteremia or anatomic splenectomy, or concerns for *ACS* (acute chest syndrome; see *Sickle Cell Emergencies*). For all patients, social issues such as an unreliable family, poor telephone access, or lack of transportation need to be considered in disposition planning. If you are not admitting a patient, be sure there is a pharmacy where they can get prescribed antibiotics overnight and that family has contact numbers for follow-up.

The middle-of-the-night fever may develop or progress in patients already in-house. Again, the initial evaluation is laboratory-based, with a better history and physical examination once antibiotics are ordered. This includes:

- CBC diff, retic (in patients with SCD), blood type & cross for patients who are also likely to be anemic or hemodynamically unstable, and chemistries (to be sure antibiotic dose modification isn't needed). For ill-appearing patients with/without bleeding, order a DIC screen and consider looking at peripheral smear for schistocytes as an indicator of microangiopathy;
- Blood culture (ideally before the first dose of antibiotics):
  - For patients with a central line, blood culture should be obtained **from all lumens**. The need for a peripheral blood culture is less clear and while we don't advocate peripheral blood culture when there is a perfectly easy central line to access, there may be an institutional standard of practice. A single peripheral culture can be useful in determining whether a patient has bacteremia vs. line infection;

DOI: 10.1201/9781003473701-8

- Urinalysis (microscopy, culture, and sensitivities) for children <2 years or if an older patient has dysuria, urgency, or a history of urinary tract infections. Whether to catheterize a child who can't urinate before antibiotics are started is also a bit up for grabs. **Patients with neutropenia may have a UTI without pyuria;**
- Start antibiotics stat (ordering is not the same thing as administering and sometimes reminders to nursing and pharmacy are needed). Many centers agree that antibiotics should be administered **within 60 minutes of presentation**.
  - For neutropenic patients (don't stand on ceremony for the child with cancer who has an ANC not yet below 500/mm³ but in whom you can expect a further drop over the next day or so based on the timing of past chemotherapy), broader spectrum antibiotics with pseudomonas coverage should be given: cefepime IV q 8hr with or without vancomycin. **If you are not sure and give ceftriaxone first, follow it with cefepime (50 mg/kg max 2 g for both cefepime and ceftriaxone);**
  - For non-neutropenic patients, ceftriaxone IV or IM is a good way to start. Maybe order 2 days' worth and in the light of day, decide on the duration of therapy;
- Patients with SCD have an increased risk of sepsis from polysaccharide-encapsulated organisms such as *Pneumococcus*, *Salmonella*, *Hemophilus Influenzae* type B, and *Escherichia coli*. Even if a patient has been on penicillin prophylaxis and is up to date on pneumococcal and *Hemophilus* vaccinations, fever in SCD is still considered an emergency due to the possibility of penicillin-resistant organisms (see *Sickle Cell Emergencies*). **Some centers** (not ours) **advise against ceftriaxone in SCD** since it can cause fatal immune hemolytic anemias and gallstones. Refinements in antibiotics (e.g., the addition of vancomycin for resistant *Strep pneumoniae*, or anaerobic coverage such as metronidazole, change in dosing for meningitis) may be needed overnight, based on serial history and physical examination:
  - A comprehensive history which we won't belabor here needs to document potential sources of fever and severity of illness, presence of central lines, drug allergies that might change antibiotic management;
  - Physical exam to look for sources of fever and assess patient stability needs to be comprehensive, including VS, weight, complete skin exam for lesions including septic emboli, *cellulitis*, perirectal lesions, look at all line sites (central lines, G-tubes, etc.). Even if you had examined the patient earlier in the day, serial **reexamination** is key if there is a change in status;
- CXR in the presence of respiratory signs and symptoms (*Acute Chest Syndrome*);
- For children with SCD, osteomyelitis that can be multifocal and that can cause fever and bone pain (that, unlike pain in most pain crises, is exquisitely point tender) should be considered and trigger orders for bone imaging (start with plain X-rays). Antibiotics in febrile patients, especially if ill-appearing patients probably shouldn't wait for needle aspiration of bone lesions. If toxic-appearing, add vancomycin (20 mg/kg once [max 2 g] and talk with the pharmacy about subsequent doses) for resistant *Strep pneumoniae*;
- IV fluids if the patient is not hemodynamically stable.

Bibliography

Lehrnbecher T, Robinson P, Fisher B, et al. Guidelines for the management of fever and neutropenia in pediatric patients with cancer and hematopoietic cell transplantation recipients. *J Clin Oncol.* 2023;41:1774–1785.

Sobota A, Sabharwal V, Fonebi G, Steinberg M. How we prevent and manage infection in sickle cell disease. *Br J Haematol.* 2015;170:757–767.

What ChatGPT Says

After lots of talk about possible etiologies, ChatGPT boiled recommendations down to: "Treatment of fever in immune-compromised patients depends on the underlying cause. It may involve antimicrobial therapy, antiviral medications, or other targeted treatments based on the specific diagnosis." A bit better when asked specifically about fever in SCD, ChatGPT is still too vague for the night-time emergency on-call:

1. *Immediate evaluation*:
   a. *Clinical assessment*: … taking a detailed medical history and performing a physical examination. This assessment should consider the patient's age, specific type of SCD (e.g., HbSS, HbSC), and underlying health status.
   b. *Temperature measurement*: Measure the patient's body temperature. Fever in adults is typically defined as a body temperature above 100.4°F (38°C).
   c. *Infection evaluation*: Determine the source of the fever, assess for potential infections, and look for specific signs and symptoms, such as pain, cough, shortness of breath, or abdominal pain, that may indicate the presence of an infection.
   d. *Blood tests*: CBC and blood cultures.

2. *Management*:
   Management of fever in individuals with sickle cell disease involves addressing the underlying cause, providing supportive care, and monitoring for complications:
   a. *Treatment of infection*: If an infection is identified, initiate appropriate antibiotic therapy. The choice of antibiotics should consider common pathogens in patients with SCD, including *Salmonella* and *Streptococcus pneumoniae*. Empirical antibiotics are often started while awaiting culture results.
   b. *Pain management*: Fever may exacerbate sickle cell pain crises. Address any pain or discomfort promptly with analgesics and supportive care.
   c. *Hydration*: Ensure the patient stays well-hydrated to prevent dehydration, which can contribute to sickle cell crises.
   d. *Oxygen*: Patients with severe respiratory symptoms may require supplemental oxygen therapy.
   e. *Hospitalization*: Depending on the severity of the infection, fever, or complications, individuals with SCD may need hospitalization for close monitoring and intravenous therapy.

    f. *Transfusions*: In some cases, blood transfusions may be necessary to treat complications such as acute chest syndrome, which can be triggered by infections.

    g. *Close monitoring*: Frequent clinical assessments, vital sign monitoring, and repeat laboratory …

Algorithm: Fever in High-Risk Populations (A)

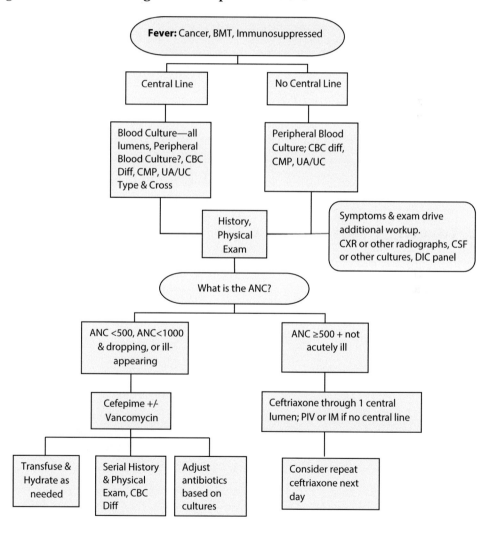

Algorithm: Fever in High-Risk Populations (B)

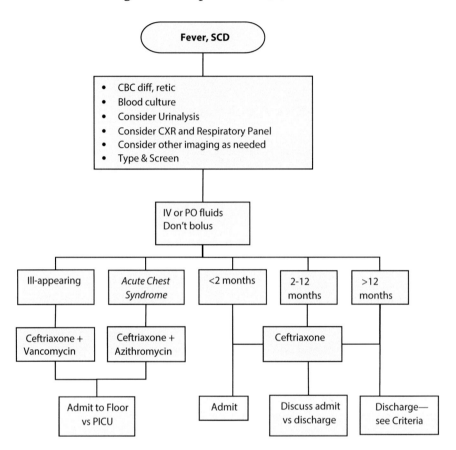

8

Typhlitis

Typhlitis, or ileocecitis, refers to inflammation of the cecum or adjacent small bowel which can lead to perforation, toxic megacolon, sepsis, and death. It looks a whole lot like appendicitis with right lower quadrant pain, fever, nausea, vomiting, and diarrhea, and is thought to result from many factors, including prolonged neutropenia (thus its other name, neutropenic enterocolitis), alteration in gut flora and mucosal injury. The diagnosis is suspected based on this history and physical findings, especially in a patient with neutropenia. Confirmatory testing includes stat CT scan with IV contrast and findings of bowel wall thickening, pneumatosis, and ileus. Even before imaging, treatment should begin:

- Make patient NPO (nothing by mouth) for gut rest;
- Start maintenance IV fluids;
- Talk with the patient and family to tell them the plan;
- Blood culture (aerobic, anaerobic);
- Start antibiotics. Zosyn (piperacillin/tazobactam) is a great choice for Gram-negative and anaerobic coverage;
- Add PO vancomycin or IV metronidazole if C. Difficile is a consideration;
- Abdominal Xray in left lateral decubitus to assess for free air;
- Pain control ideally with non-opioid medications, since opioids may make it harder to monitor symptoms;
- Consult your surgical team to get a baseline exam and assess the need for surgical intervention.

Bibliography

Cross SJ, Patel JR, Wolf J. Diagnosis and management of Typhlitis and Neutropenic Enterocolitis in children with cancer. *Pediatr Infect Dis J*. 2022;41:41e326–e328.

What ChatGPT Says

More vague overviews.

1. *Diagnosis*:
   a. *Clinical assessment*: … Common symptoms may include abdominal pain, fever, diarrhea, and generalized malaise.
   b. *Medical history*: Information regarding the patient's underlying condition, recent treatments, and medications is essential.
   c. *Imaging studies*:
      - *Abdominal computed tomography (CT) scan*: This is the most important diagnostic tool for typhlitis. It can reveal thickening of the bowel wall, inflammation, and other characteristic findings in the cecum and colon.
   d. *Blood tests*:
      - *Complete blood count (CBC)*: Neutropenia is common in typhlitis…
      - *Inflammatory markers*: Blood tests such as C-reactive protein (CRP) and erythrocyte sedimentation rate (ESR).
2. *Management*:

   Management of typhlitis involves addressing the underlying condition and providing supportive care to prevent complications…

   a. *Discontinue or adjust chemotherapy*: In cases where chemotherapy is the underlying cause of typhlitis, it may need to be temporarily halted or adjusted…
   b. *Antibiotics*: Broad-spectrum antibiotics are often started to cover potential bacterial pathogens and prevent infection progression. The choice of antibiotics should be guided by local resistance patterns.
   c. *Supportive care*:
      - *Fluid and electrolyte management*: Adequate hydration and electrolyte balance should be maintained, especially in cases of diarrhea and fever.
      - *Pain management*: Pain relief is essential, and analgesics can be administered as needed.
      - *Nutritional support*: Patients may require parenteral nutrition (intravenous feeding) if they are unable to tolerate oral intake.
   d. *Surgical consultation*: In cases of bowel perforation, surgery may be necessary to repair the damaged bowel.
   e. *Close monitoring*: Frequent clinical assessments, vital sign monitoring, and repeat imaging studies are crucial to track the patient's progress and response to treatment.
   f. *Prevention*: Prophylactic antibiotics may be considered in high-risk patients to prevent typhlitis during chemotherapy.

Algorithm: **Typhlitis**

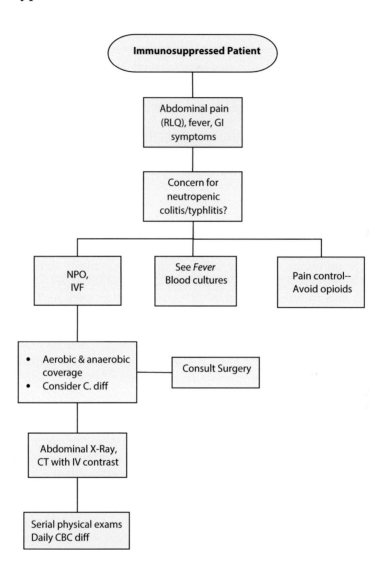

9

Methotrexate Toxicity

Methotrexate toxicity is seen almost exclusively in the setting of high-dose (HD) IV methotrexate (5–12 g/m² usually over 4 hours) or intermediate dose (3 g/m² usually over 24 hours) methotrexate as used in patients with ALL or osteosarcoma and presents either as oliguric renal failure or with methotrexate levels that are too high for COG (or another cooperative group)-determined algorithms. Methotrexate toxicity is occasionally seen with intrathecal methotrexate. The best treatment of course is prevention so that patients getting high or moderate dose methotrexate should have normal BUN and Cr levels and balanced I/O **before** starting the drug—and many centers don't start HD methotrexate after, say, 6pm to minimize nighttime chaos (Know your center's standard of practice). Monitor I/O at least every 6 hours to be sure that O $\geq$ I, and urine pH $\geq$ 7. Patients should not be on **drugs that interfere with methotrexate excretion such as TMP-SMX (septra or Bactrim), NSAIDs, penicillins, proton pump inhibitors, Lasix, or aspirin-containing medications** on the day of HD methotrexate infusion and until the methotrexate level is less than 0.4 µM (or whatever your institution recommends). Beware effusions in which methotrexate can accumulate and then be released from, causing delayed excretion. Patients should get leucovorin per protocol (usually beginning 24–30 hours from the start of methotrexate). Know what levels to expect, and when and where you can find treatment algorithms should a problem arise. One great algorithm can be found in COG AALL0434 Appendix IV but **see whatever protocol the patient is on** since the devil is in the details. **Speak with nursing** to be sure you know when leucovorin will be given and that the RN understands the parameters for calling you. Even if you were not the person to order the chemotherapy, you may be left cleaning up the mess on nights when a patient is found to have a level that is high. Ideally, you will be called with high results but realistically **be sure you know when you start call who is getting blood drawn, at what time, and track the results**—don't wait for the lab to call—set your alarm if you want to get some rest and know when to anticipate results. This is not something that should wait until AM. When levels are high, interventions are:

- Stop the methotrexate and remove/replace IV tubing through which the methotrexate was running;
- Increase the rate of IV Ringer's Lactate or D5 1/4 NS + 30 mEq/L NaHCO3 from 125 mL/m²/hr to 200 mL/m² with extra bicarb infusions as needed to maintain urine pH $\geq$ 7; consider 10–20 mL/kg fluid bolus. Alternatively, just increase IV fluids and diurese with chlorthiazide (diuril)—**no Lasix (furosemide)** with methotrexate;
- Weigh the patient serially and diurese as needed;
- Increase leucovorin to 250–1,000 mg/m² q6hr as needed, based on algorithms;

DOI: 10.1201/9781003473701-10

- For very high levels (algorithms will guide you), think about glucapardase (carboxypeptidase or Voraxaze®), which should decrease methotrexate levels by 98% within minutes, repeat levels and continue leuovorin for at least 48 hr post glucapardase. Most of the follow-up will happen on successive days;
- Watch for complications of HD methotrexate including *posterior reversible encephalopathy syndrome (PRES)*.

Bibliography

Leung KKY, Hon KL, Hui WF, et al. Therapeutics for paediatric oncological emergencies. *Drugs Context*. 2021;10:1–12.

What ChatGPT Says

Not much and not enough.

Methotrexate toxicity can occur due to overdosage, impaired drug elimination, or interactions with other medications. It can lead to serious side effects, such as bone marrow suppression, liver dysfunction, and renal impairment. Here are the key steps in diagnosing and managing methotrexate toxicity:

1. *Diagnosis*:
   a. *Clinical assessment*: … clinical assessment, including a detailed medical history and physical examination. They should inquire about the patient's methotrexate regimen, including dose, frequency, and any recent changes.
   b. *Methotrexate levels*: Measurement of serum methotrexate levels is a key diagnostic tool…
   c. *Laboratory tests*:
      - Complete blood count (CBC).
      - Liver function tests.
      - Renal function tests.
   d. *Imaging studies*: In certain cases, imaging studies, such as liver ultrasound or liver biopsy, may be performed to evaluate for liver toxicity.
2. *Management*:
   Management of methotrexate toxicity involves reducing the drug's concentration in the body, supporting organ function, and preventing further harm:
   a. *Discontinue methotrexate*: The first step is to halt methotrexate administration to prevent further exposure.
   b. *Hydration and urinary alkalinization*: Intravenous hydration with normal saline and urinary alkalinization with sodium bicarbonate can help enhance methotrexate elimination through the kidneys.

   c. *Leucovorin Rescue*: Leucovorin (folinic acid) is often administered to counteract the toxic effects of methotrexate. It provides cells with an alternative form of folate that bypasses the metabolic block caused by methotrexate. The timing, dose, and duration of leucovorin therapy depend on the severity of toxicity.

   d. *Supportive care*:
  - *Hematologic support*: Blood transfusions and growth factors (e.g., filgrastim) may be required to manage severe bone marrow suppression.
  - *Liver and renal support*: In cases of severe liver or kidney toxicity, specialized care, including dialysis or liver support, may be necessary.

   e. *Close monitoring*: Frequent clinical assessments, vital sign monitoring, and repeat laboratory tests.

   f. *Prevention*: Methotrexate dosing should follow established guidelines, and patients should be educated about the importance of adherence to dosing instructions and regular follow-up visits.

Algorithm

These are protocol-based so refer to whatever study the patient is being treated on or per. Think about identifying this **before your call** starts.

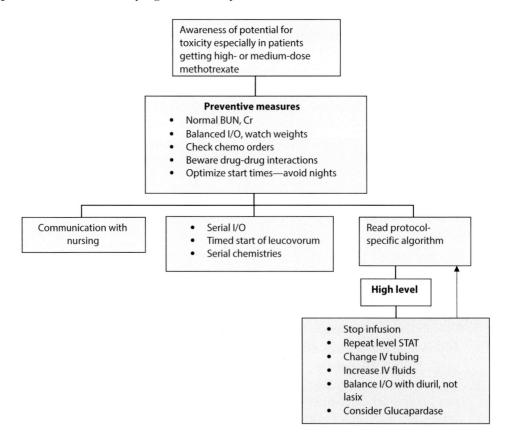

10

Posterior Reversible Encephalopathy Syndrome (PRES)

Posterior reversible encephalopathy syndrome (PRES) should be considered in a patient who exhibits acute or subacute onset of some combination of headaches, seizures, altered mental status or visual disturbances. *Methotrexate toxicity* is one of the most common reasons for PRES but it also can be caused by cyclosporine or tacrolimus as used in transplant patients, by hypertension, renal disease, or thrombotic thrombocytopenic purpura (TTP), among other problems. Suspicion is key (since patients can die from herniation or hemorrhage) and diagnosis is supported by MRI scans, which typically show changes in the posterior parietal or occipital lobes. What those changes are is best left to the neuroradiologist from whom you probably will get a wake-up call if the scan is done in the middle of the night. Vasogenic edema and even infarcts can be seen. MRI should not be done until **after you stabilize a child's airway and vital signs**. Your next intervention—if someone hasn't already done this and maybe before getting an MRI—may be to call a rapid response and consider transferring the patient to the PICU. Treatment overall is supportive care and your overnight contribution from there will be:

- To call your attending who won't want to be surprised with this the next day;
- Discontinue contributory medications—you may need to look up each of the medications a child is or recently has been on--substitutions (as for cyclosporine) can be talked about in the AM. In some cases, offending medications can be continued or reintroduced with/without dose modification;
- To control blood pressure with antihypertensive medications and seizures with antiepileptics;
- If a patient on methotrexate still has significantly high drug levels, see *Methotrexate Toxicity*.

Bibliography

Atça AÖ, Erok B, Aydogdu S. Neuroimaging findings of posterior reversible encephalopathy syndrome (PRES) following haematopoietic stem cell transplantation in paediatric recipients. *BMC Pediatr*. 2021;21:445.

DOI: 10.1201/9781003473701-11

Fidan K, Kandur Y, Ucar M, et al. Posterior reversible encephalopathy syndrome in Henoch-Schonlein Purpura and Hemolytic uremic syndrome. *J Clin Med Res.* 2016;8:544–547.
Khan RB, Sadighi ZS, Zabrowski J, et al. Imaging patterns and outcome of posterior reversible encephalopathy syndrome during childhood cancer treatment. *Pediatr Blood Cancer.* 2016;63:523–526.

What ChatGPT Says

Not bad, not that treatment-oriented, and not tailored to pediatrics. Interestingly, no specific mention of methotrexate or BMT-immunosuppressive meds as causes.

Posterior reversible encephalopathy syndrome (PRES), also known as reversible posterior leukoencephalopathy syndrome (RPLS), is a rare neurological disorder characterized by a variety of symptoms, including headaches, altered mental status, seizures, and visual disturbances. It is often associated with conditions that cause acute increases in blood pressure, such as hypertension, eclampsia (a complication of pregnancy), certain medications, or autoimmune diseases… Here are the key steps in diagnosing and managing posterior reversible encephalopathy syndrome:

1. *Diagnosis*:
   a. *Clinical assessment*: … conduct a thorough clinical assessment, including obtaining a detailed medical history and a physical examination. Symptoms of PRES can be variable and may include headache, altered mental status, seizures, visual disturbances, and focal neurological deficits.

   b. *Blood pressure measurement*: It's important to assess the patient's blood pressure, as PRES is often associated with hypertension. Both very high and very low blood pressure can be associated with PRES.

   c. *Neuroimaging*: Brain imaging, such as magnetic resonance imaging (MRI) or computed tomography (CT) scans, is essential to diagnose PRES. MRI is the preferred imaging modality and typically reveals characteristic findings of reversible edema (swelling) and abnormalities in the posterior regions of the brain.

2. *Management*:
   Management of PRES primarily involves addressing the underlying cause and controlling symptoms:
   a. *Blood pressure control*: If hypertension is identified as the underlying cause, efforts should be made to lower and stabilize blood pressure. Medications such as antihypertensives may be administered.

   b. *Seizure control*: Seizures are a common symptom of PRES. Antiseizure medications may be prescribed to control and prevent further seizures.

   c. *Medication review*: If PRES is medication-induced, such as due to immunosuppressive drugs or certain chemotherapies, the discontinuation or adjustment of the offending medications may be necessary.

d. *Supportive care*: Supportive measures, such as close monitoring, management of symptoms (e.g., headache, nausea), and control of complications, are essential.

e. *Neurology consultation*: A neurologist should be involved in the care of patients with PRES.

f. *Close monitoring*: Frequent clinical assessments and neuroimaging to assess the resolution of brain edema.

g. *Prevention*: In cases of preeclampsia or eclampsia in pregnant individuals, timely prenatal care and close monitoring during pregnancy can help prevent the development of PRES.

PRES is generally a reversible condition, and with prompt diagnosis and appropriate management, most patients recover completely. However, severe cases can lead to complications, such as cerebral hemorrhage, and may result in permanent neurological deficits. Therefore, early recognition and intervention are essential to improve patient outcomes.

Algorithm: **Posterior Reversible Encephalopathy Syndrome (PRES)**

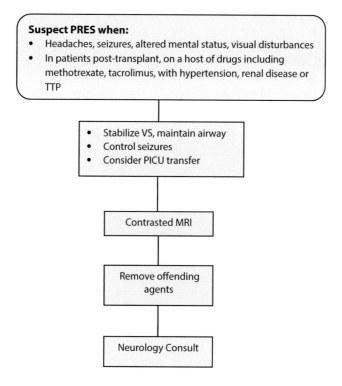

Suspect PRES when:
- Headaches, seizures, altered mental status, visual disturbances
- In patients post-transplant, on a host of drugs including methotrexate, tacrolimus, with hypertension, renal disease or TTP

- Stabilize VS, maintain airway
- Control seizures
- Consider PICU transfer

Contrasted MRI

Remove offending agents

Neurology Consult

Part II

Hematology

11

Severe Anemia

Although most of this discussion will apply to anemia of any degree, it is only the severe anemias that will be emergencies. Know normative age-dependent values for Hgb. These are available, e.g., in the Harriet Lane *Handbook* and in the Appendix of *Nathan and Oski*. The good news is that most children are not symptomatic unless the drop in Hgb from baseline is acute (over a day or so) or the anemia is severe (usually <5 g/dL). It is not unusual for children with iron deficiency from poor nutrition or slow chronic blood loss to show up in the ER with an Hgb of 4 or even 3 g/dL and feel okay. In addition, most children with severe anemia will get to a PHO (pediatric hematologist-oncologist) by way of the ER—so the initial anxiety is not on the floor. That is, unless you get a call from an outside ER or primary care doctor about a child with severe anemia. Triaging (can a consult wait a few days, does the child at home need to go to the ER first, or should he/she/they be a direct admit, or even need to be seen overnight at all?) and management will depend on your initial assessment of diagnosis and need for immediate intervention. Like many things in PHO, some laboratory studies may be available to you even before a history and physical exam. Take advantage of whatever is known already, as one of the first tenets of management is not to make the anemia worse by drawing too much blood! The basic differential is between a **bone marrow that is not producing red blood cells (RBC) with a low retic** (e.g., nutritional deficiency, *aplastic crisis* in a patient with *hemolytic anemia* such as sickle cell disease (SCD) or Thal major, primary marrow failure syndromes such as aplastic anemia, marrow replacement as with ALL) and **increased destruction usually with an elevated retic** (e.g., autoimmune *hemolytic anemia* or *splenic sequestration*). To do:

- CBC diff—is this an isolated anemia? MCV, RBC count, and MPV are all things that likely will be available by the time you hear about the patient. Ideally, you can look at a pre-transfusion peripheral smear to confirm anisocytosis (different-sized RBC) and poikilocytosis (different shapes including lots of ovalocyte-like cigar-shaped cells often in the case of iron deficiency) and not too much polychromasia (large purple RBC on smear, a surrogate for reticulocytes) and that other cell lines look okay. If you are taking call from home and the patient is being seen at your center, you will need to decide whether you need to come in to look at the slide emergently;

DOI: 10.1201/9781003473701-13

- Physical exam: vital signs and pulse oxygen level; Does the child look sick (i.e., not just pale—not to be confused with fair-skinned, and often best assessed by looking at subconjunctivae), scleral icterus, facial or other edema, hepatosplenomegaly or adenopathy, neurologic status;
- The reasonably well-appearing child with an isolated microcytic (low MCV) anemia and a low RBC count, maybe with/without thrombocytosis suggests iron deficiency (although thrombocytosis occasionally is seen in ALL and iron deficient patients can be normocytic). This often can be dealt with as an outpatient—be sure that the family has oral iron to go home with and has follow-up arranged in the PHO outpatient clinic; you can calculate a Mentzer Index but we find that this is a waste of time since mild iron deficiency and Thal syndromes usually can be differentiated just by looking at the MCV (lower in Thal trait than iron deficiency for any given Hgb and you will develop a sense for values suggesting Thal) and RBC count (higher in Thal trait than iron deficiency for any given Hgb, and Thal trait does not cause severe anemia);
  - The rare patient with a high MCV even more rarely presents as a middle-of-the-night emergency and we will ignore this for now—except if suspicion of *hemolytic anemia*;
- Fill in history: Prior heme diagnosis (SCD, Thal minor or major, *hemolytic anemia*, iron deficiency), duration of symptoms, diet (in particular how much whole cow's milk has the child been taking), bleeding history including menorrhagia (and if so, when is next period due, as menstrual bleeding may acutely lower the Hgb further); pica. Age 1–3 years old and recent infection may suggest transient erythroblastopenia of childhood (TEC) and especially in a very young child, physical dysmorphisms may suggest Diamond–Blackfan syndrome or other pure red cell aplasia;
- If the child looks sick, and ideally before, transfer to floor or PICU:
  - Add type & cross with DAT; using the least amount of blood possible, (arguably, since you may be able to make the diagnosis based on CBC and indices, you can add iron panel, ferritin, chem screen with uric acid, LDH if any suspicion of malignancy). Consider Hgb electrophoresis if previously unevaluated for hemoglobinopathy or Thal major, but again, not something you will need on nights unless you are worried about a *hemolytic transfusion reaction* in a patient with SCD;
  - If very anemic (Hgb $\leq$ 5-6g/dL) and ill-appearing, even if O_2 sat looks good, start O_2 by face mask, nasal cannula, or blow-by if the child won't tolerate anything else. **Some O_2 can be carried in plasma and may actually help alleviate symptoms**;
  - Be sure IV access is okay.
- The treatment for iron deficiency anemia generally is iron, not transfusion. If transfusion is elected in the middle of the night for patients symptomatic from anemia, see *Transfusion Emergencies*. If iron replacement is elected, start orally unless compelling reason for IV: 3–6 mg/kg/day of elemental iron. BID dosing has often given way to once-a-day dosing or even MWF dosing as adult hematology has

recommended—both because it is better tolerated and as a way to not suppress hepcidin levels and thereby to increase concomitant iron absorption. We are not sure of that in children and if iron deficiency is severe, we often still use traditional dosing divided once or twice a day. Polysaccharide iron is better tolerated and is the first choice in some centers; the use of erythropoietin is not a night-time decision;

- By the way—lead is unusual as a cause of anemia, almost never occurs before encephalopathy, but is a medical emergency—usually in this day and age handled by PICU or gen peds. If you are still worried about Pb toxicity, grab a blood level;

- If iron deficiency is suspected on the basis of menorrhagia or nose bleeds, *bleeding* evaluation can be discussed on days. If bleeding is active overnight, that may push need for transfusion, stopping periods with birth control (consider a call to GYN on-call) or epistaxis with pressure or ENT help, antifibrinolytics (tranexamic acid or amicar—see *Hemophilia*), with follow-up dosing for discussion in the morning. If patient is not too anemic, grab a PT/INR, PTT as a screen.

Bibliography

Powers JM, Buchanan GR, Adix L, et al. Effect of low-dose ferrous sulfate vs iron polysaccharide complex on hemoglobin concentration in young children with nutritional iron-deficiency anemia: a randomized clinical trial. *JAMA*. 2017;317:2297–2304.

Brugnara C, Oski FA, Nathan DG. Diagnostic approach to the anemic patient, in: Orkin S, Fisher D, Look AT, et al., eds, *Nathan and Oski's Hematology and Oncology of Infancy and Childhood*, 8th ed., Elsevier 2015; 292–307.

What ChatGPT Says

Clearly, this is for non-medical personnel and does not address emergency issues:

1. *Diagnosis*:
   a. *Clinical assessment*: … conduct a comprehensive clinical assessment, including a detailed medical history and physical examination. They should inquire about the child's symptoms, diet, family history, and any recent illnesses or infections.
   b. *Laboratory tests*:
      - Complete blood count (CBC)…
      - Peripheral blood smear…

- *Reticulocyte count*: A low reticulocyte count suggests decreased red blood cell production, while a high count may indicate hemolysis (destruction of red blood cells).
- Iron studies…
- *Additional tests*: Depending on the clinical presentation, further investigations may include serum ferritin, vitamin B_{12}, and folate levels to assess for deficiencies, as well as hemoglobin electrophoresis or genetic testing in cases of hemoglobinopathies (e.g., sickle cell anemia, thalassemia).

c. *Identifying the underlying cause*: A thorough evaluation is needed to determine the underlying cause of the anemia, which could be due to nutritional deficiencies, chronic diseases, hemolysis, or genetic conditions.

2. *Management*:

Management of severe anemia in children depends on the underlying cause and the severity of the condition. Treatment may include the following:

a. *Treating the underlying cause*:

- *Iron supplementation*: For iron-deficiency anemia, oral iron supplementation is often prescribed. In some cases, intravenous iron may be required.
- *Vitamin or folate supplementation*: For megaloblastic anemia, supplementation with vitamin B_{12} or folic acid is necessary.
- *Infections and inflammatory conditions*: Addressing and treating infections and inflammatory conditions that may be causing anemia.

b. *Blood transfusion*: In cases of severe anemia with life-threatening symptoms or complications, a blood transfusion may be necessary to rapidly improve oxygen delivery to tissues.

Algorithm: **Severe Anemia**

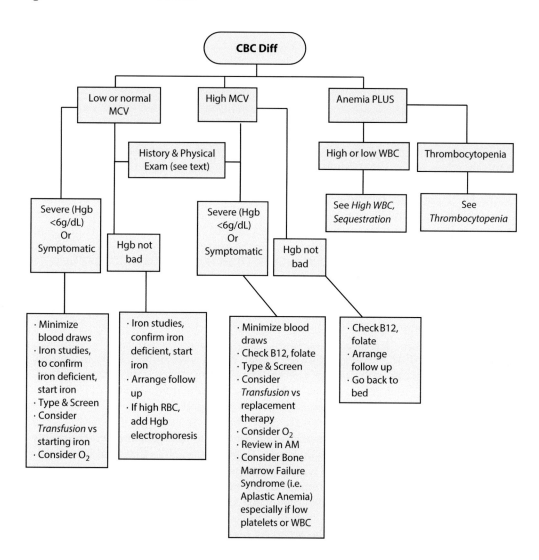

12

Hemolytic Anemia (HA)

Hemolysis refers to the breakdown of red blood cells which often is inadequately compensated for by bone marrow production, leading to anemia. The severity can range from mild (and in some cases, patients may not be anemic at all) to severe. HA can be caused by intrinsic defects (genetic/heritable conditions including enzymopathies, hemoglobinopathies, and membranopathies) or by extrinsic triggers of red cell damage, including infections, medications, mechanical shearing as through artificial valves, and/or an associated oncologic process. As with sickle cell disease (SCD) **all HA can be complicated by red cell aplasia (aplastic crises) or by splenic sequestration**. Emergency evaluations will be dictated by the severity of the anemia (patients can be clinically unstable especially if hemolysis is of acute onset) and by the time you hear about the problem, laboratory studies will likely be the starting point:

- CBC diff, pre-transfusion peripheral smear which you should look at yourself at some point for spherocytes (hereditary spherocytosis [HS], warm agglutinin HA), RBC inclusions, target/sickle cells, red cell fragmentation (*Thrombotic Microangiopathy*) and polychromasia that is a surrogate for the reticulocyte count that may take more time to result. See *Neonatal Hematologic Emergencies*, but peripheral smears in neonates can be more difficult to interpret and even normally have lots of anisocytosis or poikilocytosis. **Some HA**, such as that seen with G6PD deficiency, **can be intermittent with normal peripheral blood smears in-between** episodes of hemolysis. Most are normocytic normochromic but HS can be microcytic and patients usually have an elevated mean corpuscular hemoglobin concentration (MCHC). Although hemolysis usually drives the marrow to produce increased numbers of retics, **this can take a few days to rev up and may be normal at first presentation. Concurrent nutritional deficiencies** such as of iron also may interfere with retic production. Other cell lines usually but not always are normal; Type & Screen and DAT; (positivity tells you it's an underlying autoimmune process); the blood bank will tell you if there are warm or cold agglutinins which usually but not always correspond to IgG- or IgM-mediated, respectively. Other supportive labs are increased indirect bilirubin, serum transaminases, and LDH, and decreased haptoglobin (haptoglobin may be low in normal babies and in some Black Americans); mycoplasma is a relatively common cause of cold agglutinins and serologies may be helpful;

DOI: 10.1201/9781003473701-14

- History including past HA episodes going back to the newborn period, recent illness, vaccinations, icterus, dark (cola or tea-colored) urine, B symptoms including night sweats and weight loss, family history of HA, gallstones or splenectomies in patients or first-degree family members; Travel may suggest infections such as malaria that can cause episodic hemolysis;
- Physical exam with vital signs and pulse ox. Look for pallor (subconjunctivae), jaundice (conjunctivae, gums, palms), and splenomegaly.

Treatment will depend on the underlying etiology, but night-time emergency management will usually only be an issue for severe cases. After laboratory studies have been sent, the first issue will be whether or not to transfuse (see *Transfusion Emergencies* and *Sickle Cell Emergencies*). Coombs+ HAs (sometimes associated with thrombocytopenia or even neutropenia in Evans Syndrome) often respond to immunosuppressive therapy such as steroids (maybe start with IV methylprednisolone 2 mg/kg bid for several weeks followed by a prolonged taper). In cases refractory to steroids, we turn to agents like rituximab, but that's a conversation for the day team or outpatient clinic. Severe cases of autoimmune HA may require exchange transfusions to reduce antibodies in the plasma, although this rarely is arranged after hours. **And don't forget to use warmed blood for patients with cold-agglutinin disease**—you may need to hunt down a blood warmer.

Bibliography

Noronha SA. Acquired and congenital hemolytic anemia. *Pediatr Rev*. 2016;37:235–246.
Scheckel CJ, Go RS. Autoimmune hemolytic anemia: diagnosis and differential diagnosis. *Hematol Oncol Clin North Am*. 2022;36:315–324.

What ChatGPT Says

Way too general and not targeted at emergencies with new admissions. Splenectomies are not generally requested overnight…

1. *Diagnosis*:
   a. *Clinical assessment*: Healthcare providers should conduct a thorough clinical assessment…. inquire about the child's symptoms, growth, development, and any family history of anemia or related conditions.
   b. *Laboratory tests*:
      - *Complete blood count (CBC)*: …
      - *Blood smear*: A peripheral blood smear can reveal abnormal red blood cell morphology, including spherocytes (seen in hereditary spherocytosis) or schistocytes (seen in microangiopathic hemolytic anemias).

- *Hemolysis markers*: … lactate dehydrogenase (LDH), bilirubin levels, and haptoglobin levels to assess the degree of hemolysis.
- *Hemoglobin electrophoresis*: To rule out hemoglobinopathies like sickle cell anemia and thalassemias.
- *Reticulocyte count*: Elevated reticulocyte counts indicate increased red blood cell turnover and production.
- *Coombs test (direct and indirect)*: To determine whether the anemia is immune-related (immune hemolytic anemia).

  c. *Identifying the underlying cause*: A thorough evaluation is needed to determine the specific cause of the hemolytic anemia, which could be due to various factors, including genetic conditions, autoimmune disorders, infections, or medication-induced hemolysis.

2. *Management*:

Management of hemolytic anemia in children focuses on addressing the underlying cause, managing symptoms, and providing supportive care:

  a. *Treating the underlying cause*:

- For autoimmune hemolytic anemia, corticosteroids or other immunosuppressive medications may be prescribed.
- For hereditary conditions (e.g., hereditary spherocytosis or G6PD deficiency), specific management approaches may include splenectomy or avoiding triggers that exacerbate hemolysis.
- For infections causing hemolysis, appropriate antimicrobial therapy is required.

  b. *Blood transfusions*: In severe cases of hemolysis with symptomatic anemia, blood transfusions may be necessary to raise hemoglobin levels and improve symptoms.

  c. *Folate supplementation*: Some children may require folate supplementation, especially in cases of chronic hemolysis.

  d. *Splenectomy*: In certain hereditary hemolytic anemias, the removal of the spleen (splenectomy) may be considered to reduce the destruction of red blood cells.

  e. *Supportive care*: Supportive measures, such as pain management, hydration, and monitoring for complications (e.g., gallstones), are essential.

Algorithm: **Hemolytic Anemia**

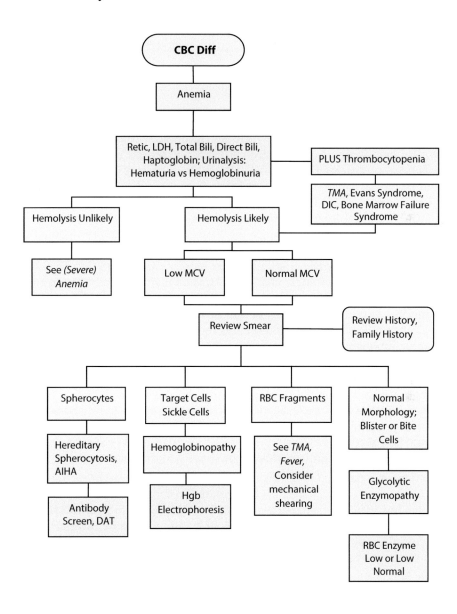

13

Thrombotic Microangiopathy (TMA)

Thrombotic Microangiopathy (TMA) includes thrombotic thrombocytopenic purpura (TTP), atypical hemolytic uremic syndrome (HUS not related to infection with *E. Coli*), and shigella toxin-producing *E. Coli* (STEC-HUS). These are true emergencies. Rapid intervention can be life-saving and is different for each of these disorders (for other causes of microangiopathy, see *Fever in High-Risk Populations* and *Bleeding Emergencies*). 70% of cases of aHUS and STEC-HUS are in children <5 years of age, and diagnosis requires high suspicion, often with serial evaluations since the characteristic thrombocytopenia (<150,000/mm^3 or a drop from baseline if one is available) and schistocytes **may not be present initially**. Patients often seek medical attention for bloody diarrhea (STEC-HUS but also in TTP), seizures, or other neurologic changes. Occasionally, a referral is from the lab calling with concerns about schistocytes (which can be seen in other microangiopathies or in small numbers in normal people). TTP can be acquired (due to autoantibodies against ADAMTS13 often following a viral illness) or is rarely congenital (Upshaw–Schulman syndrome). Evaluation includes:

- History: ask about bleeding, bruising, icterus including in the newborn period, bloody diarrhea, abdominal pain, dark urine, headaches or change in mental status; Past h/o transplant, medications including tacrolimus, cyclosporine, VEGF and checkpoint inhibitors (the list is long and you may have to look up each drug a patient is or recently has been on), family history of TMA or symptoms that suggest TMA including family members who have had dialysis;

- Laboratory evaluation: CBC diff, LFTs including Total and Direct bilirubin, stat LDH (often disproportionately high compared to drops in Hgb), haptoglobin levels (often low in normal newborns and some normal Black individuals so not diagnostic of intravascular hemolysis), CMP. **BUN and Cr can be normal even with HUS initially**; urinalysis for protein and hematuria; type & cross and DAT (which should be negative); stool culture/PCR for STEC and Shiga toxin;

  - This is one time when you and the lab tech should look at peripheral blood smear emergently—be sure to ask the lab to pull a smear stat, though initially schistocytes may be rare;

  - Once you have a strong suspicion of TMA, draw **pre-treatment pre-transfusion blood for ADAMTS 13 and anti-ADAMTS 13 antibody levels—these may not result for several days but don't forget to follow up on these** (see Algorithm);

  - Since bleeding can be seen, see evaluations for *Bleeding Emergencies…* but PT and PTT usually are normal or only incidentally abnormal;

  - **Vitamin B$_{12}$ deficiency can mimic TTP**, so consider checking B$_{12}$ and homocysteine levels;

DOI: 10.1201/9781003473701-15

- Physical examination: Vital signs are key to looking for hypertension and baseline weight; mucocutaneous bleeding, edema;
- Call transfusion medicine or renal on-call both for help with diagnosis and to arrange plasma exchange if TTP is likely (whoever does this at your center)—this should be **started based on suspicion of pending ADAMTS13 levels**;
- Call renal on-call as a heads-up even if dialysis is not needed immediately;
- Treatment includes:
  - Transfusions with PRBC or platelets as needed. A bit arbitrarily unless a patient has symptoms, consider transfusing for Hgb $\leq$7 g/dL. **Avoid platelet transfusions** unless bleeding and plt $\leq$20,000/mm^3 or for a procedure and <50,000/mm^3. Peritoneal catheter placement usually doesn't require platelet transfusion;
  - Consider plasma exchange ("plexing") **as soon as a diagnosis of TTP is suspected** to prevent ongoing vascular and organ damage;
  - Consider immunosuppression, such as steroids or rituximab. Many centers use high-dose steroids in addition to or while waiting for plasma exchange—high-dose methylprednisolone (10 mg/kg/day for 2–3 days and then 2.5 mg/kg/day until platelets >150,000/mm^3);
  - FFP in patients determined to have the congenital form of aHUS;
  - Eculizumab for aHUS, caplacizumab for TTP in adults and maybe older teens, but not for overnight; other monoclonal antibodies may be standard of care at your institution by the time this guidebook is published;
  - Try to avoid antibiotics and NSAIDs in patients with diarrhea and STEC, as this can promote HUS;
  - Limit anti-motility drugs for pain in STEC;
  - Hydrate with isotonic fluids but avoid overhydration;
  - Better definition of etiology—also may do better on morning rounds. There is a big differential diagnosis.

Bibliography

Fakhouri F, Fila M, Hummel A, et al. Eculizumab discontinuation in children and adults with atypical hemolytic-uremic syndrome: a prospective multicenter study. *Blood*. 2021;137:2438–2449.

Laurence J, Haller H, Mannucci PM, et al. Atypical hemolytic uremic syndrome (aHUS): essential aspects of an accurate diagnosis. *Clin Adv Hematol Oncol*. 2016;14(Suppl 11):2–15.

Palma LMP, Vaisbich-Guimarães MH, Sridharan M, et al. Thrombotic microangiopathy in children. *Pediatr Nephrol*. 2022;37:1967–1980.

Scully M, Goodship T. How I treat thrombotic thrombocytopenic purpura and atypical haemolytic uraemic syndrome. *Br J Haematol*. 2014;164(6):759–766.

What Chat GPT Says

Good as far as it goes. Not enough detail.

TMA includes conditions like thrombotic thrombocytopenic purpura (TTP) and hemolytic-uremic syndrome (HUS). Prompt diagnosis and management are critical to prevent complications. Here are the key steps in diagnosing and managing thrombotic microangiopathy:

1. *Diagnosis*:
   a. *Clinical assessment*: Healthcare providers should conduct a thorough clinical assessment, including obtaining a detailed medical history and performing a physical examination. Symptoms may include fatigue, weakness, pallor, petechiae, purpura, jaundice, kidney dysfunction, neurologic symptoms, and gastrointestinal symptoms.
   b. *Laboratory tests*:
      • *Complete blood count (CBC)*: This typically reveals microangiopathic hemolytic anemia (elevated reticulocyte count, schistocytes), thrombocytopenia (low platelet count), and characteristic changes in red blood cell morphology.
      • *Peripheral blood smear*: A blood smear may show schistocytes (fragmented red blood cells) and other abnormalities.
      • *Coagulation profile*: Assess for coagulation abnormalities such as elevated D-dimer levels.
      • *Renal function tests*: Assess kidney function using serum creatinine and blood urea nitrogen (BUN).
      • *LDH, bilirubin, and haptoglobin levels*: These tests can indicate the extent of hemolysis.
      • *ADAMTS13 activity*: Measuring the activity of ADAMTS13, a specific enzyme, is crucial for diagnosing TTP. Severe deficiency of ADAMTS13 activity is characteristic of acquired TTP.
   c. *Urinalysis*: Detecting blood and protein in the urine may indicate kidney involvement.
   d. *Identifying the underlying cause*: Determining the underlying cause of TMA is crucial, as it can be associated with various conditions, including TTP, HUS, autoimmune diseases, infections, and medication-induced TMA.

2. *Management*:
   Management of thrombotic microangiopathy depends on the underlying cause and severity of the condition:
   a. *Plasmapheresis (TTP)*: For acquired TTP, plasmapheresis (also known as plasma exchange) is the primary treatment. It involves removing and replacing the patient's plasma to remove autoantibodies against ADAMTS13. Plasma exchange helps restore ADAMTS13 activity and resolve the condition.
   b. *Eculizumab (Atypical HUS)*: For atypical hemolytic uremic syndrome (aHUS) caused by complement factor abnormalities, eculizumab, a complement inhibitor, may be used to prevent further complement-mediated damage.
   c. *Treatment of underlying conditions*: In cases of secondary TMA, treating the underlying cause is essential. This may involve discontinuing offending medications, managing autoimmune disorders, and treating infections.
   d. *Supportive care*: Supportive measures, including blood transfusions to correct anemia and thrombocytopenia, pain management, and kidney function support, are essential.

e. *Close monitoring*: Frequent clinical assessments, monitoring of laboratory parameters (e.g., complete blood count, renal function), and response to treatment are important to track the patient's progress.

f. *Consultation with specialists*: Consultation with hematologists, nephrologists, and other specialists may be required.

Algorithm: **Thrombotic Microangiopathy (TMA)**

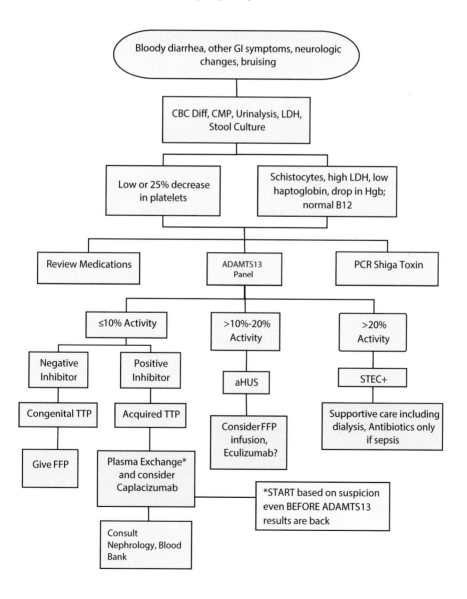

14

Transfusion Emergencies

For patients on chemotherapy, undergoing bone marrow transplantation (and for 1–2 years post-bone marrow transplant (BMT) by which time immune reconstitution usually will have occurred), newborns, or other immunosuppressed patients, blood products should be **leukoreduced** to decrease the chance of CMV transmission, alloimmunization, and non-hemolytic transfusion reactions. Leukoreduction is NOT a universal precaution and at your institution may need to be added to blood bank transfusion orders. At night, it may be easiest to order leukoreduction for all patients and rethink in the morning. This is different from **irradiated blood** products in which residual WBC are prevented from dividing and causing GVHD (see next). Indications and contraindications for transfusions for specific disorders are addressed in other sections (*High White Blood Cell Count, Severe Anemia*, TTP, *Sickle Cell Emergencies, Bleeding Emergencies*). **ABO typing generally is required for red cell transfusions but not for platelets or the rare granulocyte transfusion outside of the newborn period** (*Neonatal Hematologic Emergencies*), even when patients previously have been transfused. Rh typing should be available for all patients, and Rh-negative females who receive Rh-positive blood products (or deliver Rh-positive babies) should be given Rhogam. For a summary of what blood products have what components of the clotting system, see *Hemophilia, Von Willebrand Disease*, and *Other Factor Deficiencies*.

Special patient populations:

Sickle cell disease: Patients with sickle cell disease are at an increased risk of acute/ delayed hemolytic transfusion reactions due to incomplete cross matching and allo-immunization. Blood products should undergo extended crossmatching ("Phenotyping") for C, E, and K antigens and be sickle cell (Hgb S, C) negative. Since phenotyping and obtaining phenotyped blood products may take several hours, a "best-matched" blood product may be needed for emergencies. Sometimes phenotyping will have been done at another facility but results should be available through your blood bank.

Oncology: All immunocompromised patients **must** receive irradiated blood products to reduce the risk of transfusion-associated GVHD. This includes: Cryoglobulin (10 mL/kg—the blood bank will determine how many bags of cryo are needed to get this); fresh frozen plasma (FFP, 10 mL/kg); PRBCs (10–15 mL/kg unless it's a special patient population (e.g., see *SC Emergencies* for additional recs). Every 10 mL/kg PRBCs should raise the Hgb by ~3 g/dL.

Transfusion reactions, while only occasionally life-threatening, often occur on nights, so these are worth knowing about. Types of transfusion reactions (and these can overlap) are:

Hives/mild allergic reaction is characterized by hives but no other allergic findings (i.e., no wheezing, angioedema, or hypotension);

DOI: 10.1201/9781003473701-16

Anaphylaxis: Any allergic reaction other than hives can be part of an anaphylactic transfusion reaction. This includes angioedema, wheezing, vomiting, and/or hypotension (also seen in sepsis);

Febrile Non-Hemolytic Transfusion Reaction (FNTHR) is characterized by fever (increase in temperature $\geq 1°C$ and at least $38°C$), sometimes accompanied by chills, in the absence of other systemic symptoms;

Acute Hemolytic Transfusion Reactions (AHTR) caused by acute intravascular hemolysis of transfused red blood cells occur during or within hours of a transfusion and can be life-threatening;

Delayed Hemolytic Transfusion Reactions occur days to weeks following a transfusion with signs and symptoms similar to acute hemolytic transfusion reactions—the **key symptoms** of **acute and delayed hemolytic transfusion reactions** are progressive anemia, back pain, dark urine, and increasing jaundice. This can mimic a pain crisis in sickle cell disease (SCD) patients so **ask about transfusions within the past 21 days in patients with SCD.**

Sepsis is caused by transfusion of a product that is contaminated by a microorganism. Initial findings overlap those of febrile and hemolytic reactions and may include fever, chills, and hypotension;

Transfusion-Related Acute Lung Injury (TRALI): Life-threatening form of acute lung injury that occurs when recipient neutrophils are activated by the transfused product in an appropriately primed pulmonary vasculature;

Transfusion-Associated Circulatory Overload (TACO): is a fancy term for pulmonary edema due to volume overload.

Management of transfusion reactions centers on suspicion. A quick history and physical exam in the context of current or recent transfusions should focus on changes in vital signs (fever, tachycardia, hypo- or hypertension, respiratory distress or decreased pulse oxygenation), increasing icterus or pallor, peripheral edema. Emergency evaluations should include:

- Stop the transfusion but save the bag;
- Be sure VS are stable;
- For mild allergic reaction or fevers, you may not have to send labs. Otherwise:
- CBC, retic (even with acute hemolysis, an increase in retic may not occur immediately and can take a few days);
- Bilirubin (Total and Indirect), Cr;
- Repeat type & screen and DAT (direct Coombs test) to look for antibody formation;
- Urinalysis for hemoglobinuria;
- Recheck the transfusion product against the patient ID band to be sure the right patient got the right stuff (sounds obvious but it happens);
- Hemolytic reaction in SCD patients—resend Hgb electrophoresis/thalassemia profile to assess Hgb S and Hgb A levels if the patient is on an exchange program; Hgb A_1 levels will be lower than expected post-transfusion in the face of hemolysis;

- If there is concern for sepsis and possibly even with less suspicious febrile transfusion reactions—blood culture and culture bag containing the transfused product, and give antibiotics (see *Fever in High-Risk Populations*);
- Notify the blood bank. They may want you to send the bag back.

Bibliography

Patel RM, Josephson C. Neonatal and pediatric platelet transfusions: current concepts and controversies. *Curr Opin Hematol.* 2019;26:466–472.

Tobian A. *Approach to the patient with a suspected acute transfusion reaction.* Kleinman, S, Tirnauer, J, Waltham, MA: UpToDate Inc. Accessed on November 8, 2023.

Wang Y, Sun W, Wang X, et al. Comparison of transfusion reactions in children and adults: a systematic review and meta-analysis. *Pediatr Blood Cancer.* 2022;69:e29842.

What ChatGPT Says

Not bad, and there is considerable overlap with our overview!

1. *Acute Hemolytic Transfusion Reaction (AHTR):*
   a. *Definition*: AHTR occurs when a patient receives blood that is incompatible with their own blood type (ABO or Rh incompatibility). This can lead to rapid destruction of red blood cells, causing symptoms such as fever, chills, chest or back pain, hemoglobinuria, and shock.
   b. *Management*:
      - Stop the transfusion immediately.
      - Supportive care, including fluid resuscitation and treatment for shock, may be necessary.
      - Notify the blood bank and request a new blood unit that is compatible with the patient's blood type.
      - Identify the source of the incompatibility and take corrective actions to prevent future occurrences.
2. *Febrile Non-Hemolytic Transfusion Reaction (FNHTR):*
   a. *Definition*: FNHTR is characterized by fever during or after a transfusion, without evidence of hemolysis or other reactions. It is usually caused by recipient antibodies against donor leukocytes or platelets.
   b. *Management*:
      - Stop the transfusion if symptoms develop.
      - Administer antipyretics (e.g., acetaminophen) to manage fever.

- If recurrent FNHTR is a problem, leukocyte-reduced blood components can be considered.

3. *Allergic Transfusion Reaction*:

   a. *Definition*: Allergic reactions to transfusions can range from mild itching and rash to severe anaphylaxis. They are often caused by recipient antibodies against allergens in the donor's plasma.

   b. *Management*:

      - Stop the transfusion if symptoms occur.
      - Administer antihistamines and, in severe cases, epinephrine and corticosteroids for anaphylaxis.
      - Pre-medicate with antihistamines for patients with a history of allergic reactions to blood products.

4. *Transfusion-Related Acute Lung Injury (TRALI)*:

   a. *Definition*: TRALI is a severe acute respiratory distress reaction that can occur during or shortly after a transfusion. It is often linked to antibodies in the donor's plasma.

   b. *Management*:

      - Stop the transfusion immediately.
      - Provide oxygen and ventilatory support as necessary.
      - Report the reaction to the blood bank and return the implicated blood unit.

5. *Transfusion-Associated Circulatory Overload (TACO)*:

   a. *Definition*: TACO occurs when a patient receives blood or blood products too rapidly, leading to fluid overload. Symptoms include respiratory distress, cough, and elevated blood pressure.

   b. *Management*:

      - Slow down or stop the transfusion.
      - Administer diuretics (e.g., furosemide) to reduce fluid overload.
      - Elevate the patient's head to assist with breathing.

6. *Bacterial contamination*:

   a. *Definition*: Transfusion with blood products contaminated with bacteria can lead to septicemia. Symptoms may include fever, chills, hypotension, and shock.

   b. *Management*:

      - Stop the transfusion immediately.
      - Provide supportive care and administer appropriate antibiotics.
      - Investigate the source of contamination to prevent future occurrences.

7. *Transfusion error (e.g., wrong blood component)*:

   a. *Management*:

      - Stop the transfusion immediately.
      - Administer supportive care as needed, depending on the nature of the error.
      - Investigate the error and take corrective actions to prevent reoccurrence.

Algorithm: **Transfusion Emergencies**

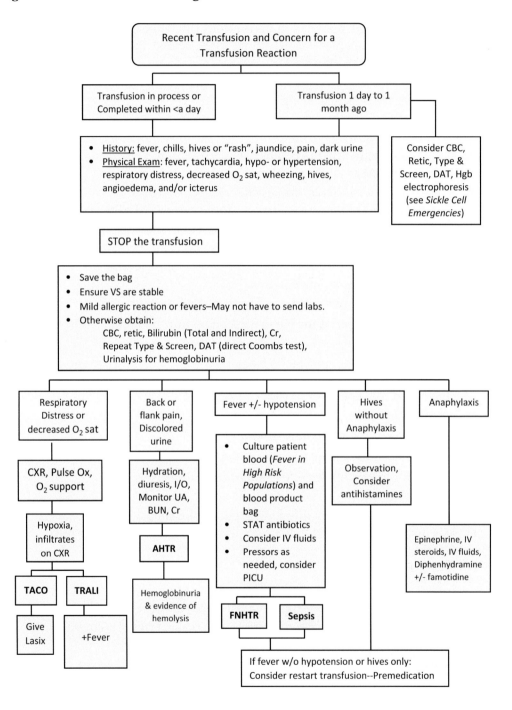

15

Sickle Cell Emergencies

These often overlap and more than one type of "crisis" can occur at a time. Almost all come through an ER but you likely will get a call. A few steps will let you know which crisis or crises are in play. Specific crises are discussed below.

- History—confirm the type of SCD (SS, SC, S beta$^{0,+}$thal); fever; pain, increasing icterus, pallor or fatigue; respiratory or neurologic changes; types of past crises. triggering events such as infections;
- Lab tests take a while to come back so get moving with these: CBC diff, retic; consider Type & Screen, LFTS with TB/Indirect Bili, blood culture if febrile (see *Fever in High-Risk Populations* and the following sections). Compare these with past results at baseline;
- Physical exam to include vital signs, pulse oxygen level, and weight to allow dosing; check for icterus and pallor and ask the family how this compares to usual; chest exam; new flow murmurs. **Change** in hepatosplenomegaly; neuro exam; GU exam, especially in males to look for *priapism*;
- Long-term preventive measures such as hydroxyurea and ketamine are not nighttime decisions for you to make now.

Bibliography

Broderick GA. Priapism and sickle-cell anemia: diagnosis and nonsurgical therapy. *J Sex Med.* 2012;9:88–103.

DeBaun MR, Jordan LC, King AA, et al. American Society of Hematology 2020 Guidelines for sickle cell disease: prevention, diagnosis, and treatment of cerebrovascular disease in children and adults. *Blood Adv* 2020;4(8):1554–1588.

Friend A, Settelmeyer TP, Girzadas D. Acute Chest Syndrome. [Updated 2023 Feb 6]. In: StatPearls [Internet]. Treasure Island (FL): StatPearls Publishing; 2023.

Idris IM, Burnett AL, DeBaun MR. Epidemiology and treatment of priapism in sickle cell disease. *Hematology Am Soc Hematol Educ Program.* 2022;2022:450–458.

Kato GJ, Piel FB, Reid CD, et al. Sickle cell disease. *Nat Rev Dis Primers.* 2018;4:18010.

Porter M. Rapid fire: Sickle cell disease. *Emerg Med Clin North Am.* 2018;36(3):567–576.

What ChatGPT Says

We queried diagnosis and management in children with SCD for each crisis type in the chapters to follow. In general, not bad but too vague to be useful on nights, with more of a focus on chronic management.

Algorithm: **Sickle Cell Emergencies (see** *Anemia, Hemolytic Anemia***)**

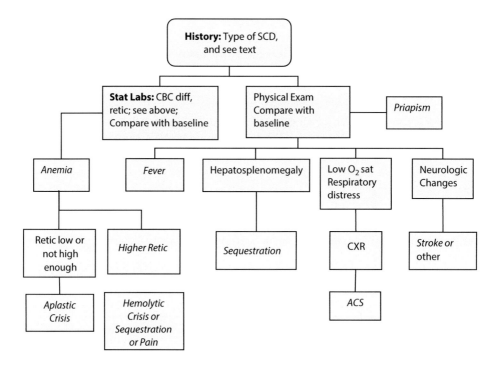

16

Acute Chest Syndrome

Acute chest syndrome (ACS) is the result of vaso-occlusion within the pulmonary vasculature of patients with SCD and is defined by a new pulmonary infiltrate on chest X-ray not likely due to atelectasis. ACS may progress quickly and is the **most common cause of death in patients with SCD. Suspicion of ACS if a child is acutely ill may be a reason for admission.** In children, infections—which also may be life-threatening—are the most common cause of ACS and most commonly are viral, mycoplasma or chlamydia pneumonias. Other causes include asthma, hypoxemia, oversedation, and post-operative complications. Patients will have some combination of chest pain, fever, tachypnea, wheezing, rales, coughing, increased work of breathing with intercostal retractions, and hypoxemia (relative to baseline). Because ACS can start insidiously and early treatment is key to successful management, a CXR is useful in patients with even modest respiratory symptoms.

- If there is *fever*, obtain a blood culture. Broad-spectrum antibiotics should be given to every child with confirmed or a strong suspicion of ACS. Third-generation cephalosporin (ceftriaxone=Rocephin) for routine bacterial coverage and a macrolide (azithromycin = Zithromax) for atypical mycobacteria—**some centers** (not ours) **advise against ceftriaxone in SCD** since it can cause fatal immune hemolytic anemias and gallstones; for patients with pen allergies, consider clindamycin or levofloxacin.
- If there is a concern for methicillin-resistant staph aureus (MRSA), vancomycin should be added. Treatment is continued for 7–10 days—but again, this discussion is just to get you through the night!
- Fluid management should be directed by the child's hydration status;
  - Avoid overhydration which can lead to pulmonary edema and diurese as needed with Lasix;
  - Supplemental oxygen should be given to correct a low SpO_2 or PaO_2. Keep 0_2 sats > 92%;
- PRBC transfusions (*Transfusion Emergencies*) have demonstrated some efficacy in case series. However there are no randomized controlled trials evaluating PRBC transfusions vs. only supportive management in ACS;
  - Exchange transfusions are often used in severe cases of ACS (especially those in which Hgb ≥ 10 g/dL) so consider talking to your blood bank and/or PICU;
- Pain control is a balance between analgesia to prevent pain, respiratory splinting that may compound atelectasis, and oversedation which can lead to hypoventilation and hypoxia;

DOI: 10.1201/9781003473701-18

- Pain control usually starts with ibuprofen or ketorolac (Toredol) since they are nonsedating and less likely to cause hypoventilation than opioids;
- Opioids are used if pain is not adequately controlled with non-steroidal anti-inflammatory drugs (NSAIDs);
- Bronchodilators in children with ACS even without bronchospasm are used in some centers;
- Steroids have been shown to shorten the length of stay **but carry the risk of a higher rate of rebound veno-occlusive crisis (VOC) and increased risk of re-admission**; think twice before using steroids on nights;
- Incentive spirometry every 2 hours while awake to prevent atelectasis. The patient's guardian or nursing team will need to push this even overnight;
- Encourage ambulation.

What ChatGPT Says

Not bad but too vague to be useful on nights, with more of a focus on chronic management.

Acute chest syndrome (ACS) is a potentially life-threatening complication in individuals with sickle cell disease (SCD), characterized by chest pain, fever, cough, and signs of lung inflammation. ACS is often triggered by vaso-occlusion in the pulmonary vessels and is a medical emergency… Here are the key steps in diagnosing and managing acute chest syndrome in individuals with sickle cell disease:

1. *Diagnosis*:
   a. *Clinical assessment*: … conduct a thorough clinical assessment, including … a detailed medical history and … physical examination. Symptoms may include chest pain, cough, fever, and respiratory distress. ACS should be suspected in individuals with SCD who develop these symptoms.
   b. *Chest imaging*: Chest X-rays or chest computed tomography (CT) scans are essential for diagnosing ACS. Typical findings may include lung opacities, infiltrates, and consolidation.
   c. *Laboratory tests*:
      - Complete blood count (CBC);
      - Pulse oximetry;
   d. *Infection Evaluation*: It's important to rule out other causes of respiratory symptoms, such as pneumonia or other infections.
2. *Management*:
   The management of acute chest syndrome in individuals with sickle cell disease involves addressing the underlying cause and providing supportive care to improve oxygenation and manage symptoms:
   a. *Hospitalization*: ACS is a medical emergency, and individuals with suspected or confirmed ACS should be hospitalized for close monitoring and treatment.

b. *Oxygen therapy*: Oxygen should be administered to maintain oxygen saturation levels above 92%. Supplemental oxygen helps improve oxygenation and reduce respiratory distress.

c. *Broad-spectrum antibiotics*: Empirical antibiotics are often started to treat or prevent bacterial infections, as infections can worsen ACS. The choice of antibiotics should consider local resistance patterns.

d. *Blood transfusion*: Exchange transfusion or simple transfusion may be indicated to increase oxygen-carrying capacity and reduce the percentage of sickled red blood cells. Exchange transfusion is preferred in severe cases.

e. *Pain management*: Analgesics, such as opioids, should be administered to alleviate chest pain and improve patient comfort.

f. *Hydration*: Adequate hydration is important to prevent vaso-occlusion and reduce the viscosity of sickled blood.

g. *Incentive spirometry*: Encourage deep breathing and the use of incentive spirometry to prevent atelectasis (lung collapse) and improve lung function.

h. *Consultation with specialists*: … consultation with a pediatric pulmonologist or critical care specialist may be required.

i. *Close monitoring*: Frequent clinical assessments, vital sign monitoring, and repeat imaging studies are essential to track the patient's progress and response to treatment.

Algorithm: see Chapter 15

17

Aplastic Crisis in SCD

Aplastic crisis occurs when the bone marrow temporarily stops producing RBCs, leading to a drop in Hgb. **This can occur in anyone with an underlying hemolytic anemia** but is most common in SCD. Rarely, aplastic crises have been reported in hematologically apparently normal individuals. Infection is the usual immediate cause and parvovirus B19 is the most talked about agent. However, other viruses and bacterial infections also can cause an aplastic crisis. Patients present with the signs and symptoms of worsening anemia (pallor, lethargy). Reticulocytopenia (at least a lower absolute retic count than the patient's baseline) is confirmatory—although **patients with isolated hemolytic crises may take a few days to rev up their retic counts** so that these types of crises may be confused early on.

What ChatGPT Says

Not bad but too vague to be useful on nights, with more of a focus on chronic management.

Aplastic crisis is … characterized by a sudden and severe drop in red blood cell production (aplastic anemia), typically triggered by parvovirus B19 infection. The management of aplastic crisis in SCD involves addressing the underlying cause, providing supportive care, and, in some cases, transfusion therapy. Here are the key steps in diagnosing and managing aplastic crisis in individuals with sickle cell disease:

1. *Diagnosis*:
   a. *Clinical assessment*… clinical assessment, including obtaining a detailed medical history and performing a physical examination. Symptoms may include fatigue, pallor, weakness, and sudden-onset severe anemia.
   b. *Laboratory tests*:
      - *Complete blood count (CBC)*: Aplastic crisis is characterized by a significant decrease in hemoglobin, red blood cell count, and reticulocyte count.
      - *Blood smear*: Examination of the blood smear may reveal the absence of reticulocytes.
      - *Parvovirus B19 serology*: Blood tests for parvovirus B19 antibodies can confirm the diagnosis of parvovirus-induced aplastic crisis.

2. *Management*:
   The management of aplastic crisis in individuals with sickle cell disease involves addressing the underlying cause and providing supportive care:

DOI: 10.1201/9781003473701-19

a. *Supportive care*: Patients with aplastic crisis may require supportive care, including adequate hydration and pain management.

b. *Discontinue exchange transfusions*: If the patient is on a chronic exchange transfusion program for SCD, this may be temporarily discontinued to allow the body to recover its red blood cell production.

c. *Blood transfusion*: In severe cases with symptomatic anemia and hemodynamic instability, red blood cell transfusion may be required to improve hemoglobin levels and oxygen-carrying capacity. Cross-match compatible blood should be used.

d. *Treatment of parvovirus infection*: If parvovirus B19 infection is confirmed, specific antiviral therapy is not available, but the body usually clears the infection spontaneously. However, intravenous immunoglobulin (IVIG) may be considered in severe cases.

e. *Close monitoring*: Frequent clinical assessments, vital sign monitoring, and repeat laboratory tests are crucial to track the patient's progress and response to treatment.

Algorithm: see Chapter 15

18

Hemolytic Crisis in SCD

Hemolytic crisis usually pairs a dropping Hgb with a relative increase in retic count, increasing indirect bilirubin and LDH. Haptoglobins also may drop below baseline although this is not often used in SCD management. As previously noted, it may take a few days for patients with hemolytic crises to rev up their retic counts so that these may be confused with aplastic crises and serial daily retic counts may be needed to sort this out. In patients for whom **delayed hemolytic transfusion reactions are not a consideration (and for whom transfusion may be a bad idea), transfusion or observation** with reassessment in the morning are both appropriate depending on how low the Hgb is and whether the retic count is high enough to predict recovery. Where a delayed hemolytic reaction is suspected, resend Hgb electrophoresis/thalassemia profile to assess Hgb S and Hgb A levels if a patient is on an exchange program: Hgb A_1 levels will be lower than expected post-transfusion in the face of hemolysis. Keep an eye on pulse oxygenation as a drop may signal concomitant *ACS* and/or a need to go ahead with PRBC. **Many patients with hemolytic anemias,** even for reasons other than SCD, **develop folate deficiency** since RBC folate is released into the blood with hemolysis and urinated out of the body. Dietary supplementation rarely keeps up and folate 1 mg a day is good supportive care. Erythropoietin may be a daytime discussion.

What ChatGPT Says

Not bad but too vague to be useful on nights, with more of a focus on chronic management.

Hemolytic crisis is a complication that can occur in individuals with sickle cell disease (SCD), where there is an accelerated breakdown of red blood cells, often leading to a severe drop in hemoglobin levels and worsening anemia. The management of hemolytic crisis in SCD involves addressing the underlying cause, providing supportive care, and, in some cases, blood transfusion. Here are the key steps in diagnosing and managing hemolytic crisis in individuals with sickle cell disease:

1. *Diagnosis*:
    a. *Clinical assessment*: ... conduct a thorough clinical assessment, including obtaining a detailed medical history and performing a physical examination. Symptoms may include jaundice, fatigue, pallor, dark urine, and worsening anemia.

DOI: 10.1201/9781003473701-20

b. *Laboratory tests*:

- *Complete blood count (CBC)*: Hemolytic crisis is characterized by a significant decrease in hemoglobin, hematocrit, and red blood cell count.
- *Blood smear*: Examination of the blood smear may reveal red blood cell abnormalities, such as fragmented cells (schistocytes), spherocytes, and reticulocytosis.
- *Blood chemistry*: Elevated levels of bilirubin and lactate dehydrogenase (LDH) in the blood can be indicative of hemolysis.
- *Hemoglobin electrophoresis*: To confirm the presence of SCD and rule out other hemoglobinopathies.

2. *Management*:

The management of hemolytic crisis in individuals with sickle cell disease involves addressing the underlying cause and providing supportive care:

a. *Supportive care*: Patients with hemolytic crisis may require supportive care, including pain management, hydration, and measures to prevent complications like gallstones.

b. *Identify and treat triggers*: Determine the underlying cause of the hemolysis and address it. Common triggers include infections, oxidative stress, or sickle cell-related complications.

c. *Blood transfusion*: In severe cases with symptomatic anemia, blood transfusion may be necessary to raise hemoglobin levels and alleviate symptoms. Cross-match compatible blood should be used.

d. *Management of pain*: Pain management is crucial, as hemolytic crisis can be associated with severe pain. Analgesics, including opioids, are typically administered to provide relief.

e. *Consultation with specialists*: Collaboration with a hematologist experienced in the care of patients with SCD is essential. Depending on the specific circumstances, consultations with other specialists (e.g., infectious disease specialists) may be needed.

f. *Close monitoring*: Frequent clinical assessments, vital sign monitoring, and repeat laboratory tests are necessary to track the patient's progress and response to treatment.

Algorithm: see Chapter 15

19

Pain or Vaso-occlusive Crisis in SCD

Pain or vaso-occlusive crisis can be associated with any other crisis but even if isolated, management is symptom relief balanced against respiratory suppression and alteration of mental status: fluid management to avoid dehydration, consider PRBC transfusion (*Transfusion Emergencies*) for refractory pain (although not evidence-based) and **be sure that pain isn't actually osteomyelitis**. Review medical records and ask the family what has worked in the past. Schedule analgesia (e.g., acetaminophen, ibuprofen, and/or oxycodone PO or IV q6 hr or IV ketorolac [Toradol]) with additional opioids for breakthrough pain. Have a low threshold for starting a patient-controlled analgesia (PCA) pump. Some centers quantify pain using the Wong–Baker faces rating scale.

What ChatGPT Says

Not bad but too vague to be useful on nights, with more of a focus on chronic management.

Sickle cell pain crisis, also known as a vaso-occlusive crisis, is … characterized by severe, sudden-onset pain … Here are the key steps in diagnosing and managing pain crises in individuals with sickle cell disease:

1. *Diagnosis*:
   a. *Clinical assessment*: … detailed medical history and performing a physical examination. Symptoms may include severe pain, typically in the bones or joints, but can affect any part of the body.
   b. *Pain assessment*: Healthcare providers use various pain assessment scales, such as the numerical rating scale (NRS) or the Wong–Baker FACES Pain Rating Scale, to assess the intensity and location of the pain.
   c. *Exclude other causes*: It is important to rule out other causes of pain, such as infections, bone fractures, or other complications.
2. *Management*:

   Management of a pain crisis in individuals with sickle cell disease involves several components, including pain relief, hydration, and addressing potential triggers:
   a. *Pain relief*:
      - *Analgesics*: Opioid medications, such as morphine, hydromorphone, or fentanyl, are often required for pain control. Pain medication should be administered promptly and titrated based on the individual's pain level.

DOI: 10.1201/9781003473701-21

- *Non-opioid analgesics*: Non-steroidal anti-inflammatory drugs (NSAIDs) like ibuprofen or acetaminophen may be used as adjuncts to opioids for mild to moderate pain.
- *Patient-controlled analgesia (PCA)*: In some cases, patients may be given access to a PCA pump, which allows them to self-administer pain medication within prescribed limits.

b. *Hydration*: Maintaining adequate hydration is important to help prevent further sickling of red blood cells and improve blood flow. Intravenous (IV) fluids are typically administered to ensure proper hydration.

c. *Oxygen therapy*: In some cases, supplemental oxygen is provided to help increase oxygen delivery to tissues and reduce pain.

d. *Address triggers*: Identify and address any potential triggers of pain crises, such as infections, dehydration, or exposure to extreme temperatures.

e. *Management of complications*: Pain crises can lead to complications such as acute chest syndrome or stroke. If complications arise, they should be managed promptly.

f. *Pain diary*: Encourage the patient to keep a pain diary to track the severity, location, and duration of pain episodes. This can help in tailoring the treatment plan and assessing the effectiveness of interventions.

g. *Educate* the patient and their family about SCD, pain management strategies, and when to seek medical attention.

Effective management of pain crises in SCD often involves a multi-modal approach.

Algorithm: **see Chapter 15**

20

Priapism in SCD

Priapism—prolonged penile erection often not associated with sexual stimulation—is a urologic emergency since prolonged priapism can result in impotence. It can occur at any age but is most common during adolescence. Retrospectively, priapism has been classified as "stuttering" when it resolves—often spontaneously—within 4 hours or "major/fulminant" when the duration is longer than 4 hours. In many cases, patients are not seen by a healthcare provider until erections are very prolonged so that intervention is urgent.

Initial management beyond what is listed in chapter 19 includes

- History to document duration, degree of pain, whether the erections are getting better or not, underlying diagnosis of SCD, possible inciting events such as trauma, masturbation or other sexual activity, medications, infections, urinary retention;
- Physical examination to document and characterize the erection;
- Talk with the patient and family to tell them the plan;
- If less than two hours from the onset, give IV fluids (consider **not using normal saline-containing fluids, to avoid hypertonicity**) followed by IV + PO goal of 100% maintenance rate. For more prolonged priapism give NS bolus 10–20 mL/kg followed by IV + PO goal of 100% maintenance rate;
- For Hgb $\leq$ 6 g/dL, or 2 points below baseline and/or priapism persisting beyond 4 hours and/or recurring, consider simple blood transfusion;
- Analgesia (see *Pain/Vaso-occlusive Crisis*) and anxiolytic agents such as Ativan as needed. Priapism can be very painful—ask the patient what has worked for him in the past;
- Have the patient take a warm bath and/or apply a warm compress to the penis;
- Encourage the patient to urinate and masturbate to promote detumescence;
- Order **pseudoephedrine**. Start with 0.5 mg/kg (max 60 mg) bid (for 3 days, but remember—all you have to do is get through the night before you can clarify the duration with your team). If this is successful in achieving detumescence, then it can be stopped;
- Consult the (pediatric) urologist on-call for a discussion of the need for duplex ultrasound to differentiate between high-flow (i.e., non-ischemic) and low-flow (i.e., ischemic) priapism, penile aspiration, intra-corporeal injection of phenylephrine, and washout—or various shunting procedures if none of the interventions works.

DOI: 10.1201/9781003473701-22

What ChatGPT Says

Not bad but too vague to be useful on nights, with more of a focus on chronic management.

Priapism is a painful, prolonged erection of the penis that can be a complication of sickle cell disease (SCD), specifically, sickle cell anemia. Priapism occurs when blood becomes trapped in the erectile tissue of the penis and is unable to drain properly … Here are the key steps in diagnosing and managing priapism in individuals with sickle cell disease:

1. *Diagnosis*:
   a. *Clinical assessment*: … conduct a thorough clinical assessment, including obtaining a detailed medical history and performing a physical examination. Symptoms may include persistent, painful erection unrelated to sexual stimulation.
   b. *Duration assessment*: Priapism is typically classified into two main types based on duration:
      - *Low-flow (ischemic) priapism*: The most common type associated with SCD. It is characterized by a prolonged, painful erection with decreased blood flow to the penis.
      - *High-flow (non-ischemic) priapism*: Less common and not typically associated with SCD. It is characterized by a prolonged, painless erection with normal or increased blood flow to the penis.
2. *Management*:
   Management of priapism in individuals with sickle cell disease involves several components, including pain relief and interventions to resolve the priapism:
   a. *Pain relief*: Pain management is a priority and may involve the use of analgesics, such as opioids (e.g., morphine), to alleviate the pain associated with priapism.
   b. Non-invasive measures for low-flow priapism:
      - *Hydration*: Maintaining proper hydration is important to reduce the viscosity of sickled blood and improve blood flow.
      - *Warm compresses*: Applying warm compresses to the genital area can help promote blood flow and alleviate pain.
      - *Oral medications*: Some medications, like pseudoephedrine, may be prescribed to constrict blood vessels and relieve priapism.
   c. *Aspiration and injection for low-flow priapism*:
      - *Aspiration*: A healthcare provider may use a syringe and needle to withdraw blood from the affected area, which can relieve the priapism.
      - *Phenylephrine injection*: Phenylephrine, a vasoconstrictor, may be injected directly into the penis to help alleviate priapism by constricting blood vessels.

d. *Consultation with specialists*: Collaboration with urologists and hematologists experienced in the care of patients with SCD is essential, especially for prolonged or recurrent cases of priapism.

e. *Surgical measures for high-flow priapism*: In cases of high-flow priapism, where the problem is excessive blood flow to the penis, surgical intervention may be required to correct the underlying issue. This typically involves arterial embolization.

f. *Consideration of exchange transfusion*: In some severe and prolonged cases, exchange transfusion may be considered to improve oxygen delivery and blood flow to the penis.

g. *Education*: Patients with sickle cell disease and their families should be educated about priapism, its symptoms, and the importance of seeking prompt medical attention.

Algorithm: see **Chapter 15**

21

Splenic Sequestration in SCD

Splenic sequestration refers to the pooling of blood in an enlarging spleen. This can be an acute process with dramatic sudden drops in Hgb, often drops in platelet counts, and can result in death if not addressed promptly. Sequestration can be asymptomatic but typical signs and symptoms are pallor, lethargy, abdominal pain and distension, and a spleen size bigger than baseline. Although sequestration is most commonly seen in young children (<2 years) with sickle cell disease (i.e., before they have experienced auto-infarction of their spleens) and is the second most common cause of SCD deaths in the first decade, it can occur in the setting of **any** *hemolytic anemia*. In patients who have had splenectomy, **sequestration still can occur in the liver or in accessory spleens** if these weren't removed. Sequestration usually arises in the setting of infection so that patients may be febrile. For the child who is suspected of sequestration emergency management in addition to the steps above, should include:

- Comparison of Hgb with prior "baseline" labs;
- Type & cross: Ideally this should be with "phenotyped blood" to minimize transfusion reactions, but urgency may not allow this. A call to the blood bank to give them a heads-up about urgency is a good idea. In some situations O-neg blood may be the fastest and best initial transfusion;
- The ill patient will need a minimum of every 30-min observations (heart rate, pulse rate, O_2 saturations, and blood pressure) until stabilized. This degree of monitoring may require PICU nursing;
- Give supportive oxygen therapy if O_2 sats <92% **or if very low Hgb** (e.g., 2 g/dL) is suspected, even if sats are good, in order to increase circulating O_2;
- For hemodynamically tenuous patients give fluid bolus (10 mL/kg NS or Ringer's lactate and re-evaluate in 15 minutes, repeat × 2 [total of 30 mL/kg]) within 1 hour or until BP/HR stabilizes while pressing Blood Bank to send blood;
  - When blood arrives, transfuse **5 mL/kg over 3–4 hours**. The hope is that **patients will auto-transfuse** and get to a goal Hb of 8 g/dL which often occurs without additional transfusions. Take care **not to over-transfuse** as the recovering spleen (or liver) will release pooled blood to the circulation and can lead to hyperviscosity;
- Recheck Hgb one hour after transfusion and repeat transfusion as appropriate;
- If febrile, see *Fever in High-Risk Populations*/SCD;
- Monitor spleen size for the first 12–24 hours until it starts to shrink;

DOI: 10.1201/9781003473701-23

- Discharge planning won't be a middle-of-the-night issue but remember to counsel the family about what to look for in the future and arrange outpatient pediatric hematology oncology (PHO) follow-up. **Sequestration can be a recurrent event and discussion of prophylactic splenectomy is warranted** on rounds.

What ChatGPT Says

Not bad but too vague to be useful on nights, with more of a focus on chronic management.

Splenic sequestration crisis is a serious and potentially life-threatening complication of sickle cell disease (SCD), primarily occurring in young children with the condition. This crisis is characterized by a rapid and massive enlargement of the spleen, leading to sequestration (trapping) of a large portion of blood within the spleen.

1. *Diagnosis*:
   a. *Clinical assessment*: … conduct a thorough clinical assessment, including obtaining a detailed medical history and performing a physical examination. Symptoms may include sudden and severe abdominal pain, pallor, fatigue, and signs of shock.
   b. *Laboratory tests*:
      - *Complete blood count (CBC)*: This will show a significant drop in hemoglobin levels …due to blood pooling in the spleen.
      - *Reticulocyte count*: Reticulocytosis (an increased number of immature red blood cells) may be present as the body attempts to compensate for the drop in red blood cell count.
   c. *Ultrasonography or imaging*: Ultrasonography or other imaging studies may be performed to confirm spleen enlargement and rule out other causes of abdominal pain.
2. *Management*:
   The management of splenic sequestration crisis in individuals with sickle cell disease involves addressing the underlying crisis, providing supportive care, and preventing further complications:
   a. *Hospitalization*: Splenic sequestration is a medical emergency, and individuals with this condition should be hospitalized for close monitoring and treatment.
   b. *Blood transfusion*: Transfusion of red blood cells may be necessary to raise hemoglobin levels and stabilize the patient's condition.
   c. *Supportive care*: Supportive measures, including oxygen therapy and intravenous (IV) fluids, are essential to improve oxygen delivery, maintain hydration, and support circulation.
   d. *Pain management*: Pain relief is critical, and analgesics may be administered to alleviate abdominal pain and discomfort.

e. *Monitoring*: Frequent clinical assessments, vital sign monitoring, and repeat laboratory tests are essential to track the patient's progress and response to treatment.

f. *Consultation with specialists*: Collaboration with hematologists and pediatric surgeons experienced in the care of patients with SCD is crucial, especially for severe or recurrent cases.

g. *Splenectomy*: In some cases, particularly if the patient experiences recurrent or severe splenic sequestration crises, surgical removal of the spleen (splenectomy) may be considered to prevent further crises. However, the decision to perform a splenectomy is individualized and should be carefully discussed with the healthcare team.

Algorithm: **see Chapter 15**

22

Stroke in SCD

Stroke in SCD is caused by sickled RBCs leading to vessel obstruction and ischemia in the brain. Stroke should be suspected with the onset of any **new neurological symptoms** in a patient with SCD, some of which include decreased level of consciousness, seizures, acute weakness, or paralysis of one or more limbs, severe headache, slurred speech, blurred vision, or abnormal behavior/sudden personality change. Even though similar symptoms that haven't lasted 24 hours can be considered a transient ischemic attack (TIA), in the middle of the night and for most of us at any time, such symptoms should be considered to be a stroke, which **is an emergency**. In addition to the above labs:

- Tox screen: remember to check the results. **Not everything in SCD relates to SCD**;
- If febrile, refer to *Fever in High-Risk Populations*;
- Be sure the patient is stable; i.e., airway, oxygenation, and circulation;
- Oxygen therapy to ensure oxygen saturations of >92% (if hypoxia is present, see *Acute Chest Syndrome*);
- Once the patient is stable, obtain an uncontrasted CT scan of the head to identify hemorrhagic stroke, although this is less common in children than adults with SCD, or a contrasted MRI if this can be obtained quickly;
- Arrange for emergency exchange transfusion ideally within 2 hours of recognition of acute neurological symptoms (the goal of red cell exchange is to reduce the hemoglobin S concentrations to <30%);
    - If an exchange transfusion is not an option, you can give a simple blood transfusion 10 mL/kg if Hgb $\leq$ 8 g/dL to achieve Hgb of **no more than 10 g/dL** while awaiting exchange transfusion (this may require transfer to another center if yours can't accommodate);
    - If Hgb is >8 g/dL, then arrange red cell exchange transfusion manually or automated; this may require transfer to the PICU for better IV access and generally just for help (although this doesn't mean you can forget about the patient, and PHO should remain involved);
    - Hydration with caution: The goal is euvolemia. Avoid dehydration or hyperhydration which can lead to cerebral edema;
- Consult pediatric neurology and possibly neurosurgery;
- After the exchange is complete, get a brain MRI and MRA (w/wo contrast). This may not happen for a day or so and may fall to the PICU. **Transcranial dopplers (TCD)** are not a night-time emergency, but you should review the most recent TCDs to confirm stroke risk.

DOI: 10.1201/9781003473701-24

What ChatGPT Says

Not bad but too vague to be useful on nights, with more of a focus on chronic management.

Stroke is a severe and potentially life-threatening complication of sickle cell disease (SCD), especially in children. Stroke in individuals with SCD typically results from the occlusion of blood vessels in the brain due to sickled red blood cells. Early diagnosis and management are essential to minimize neurological damage and prevent future strokes. Here are the key steps in diagnosing and managing stroke in individuals with sickle cell disease:

1. *Diagnosis*:
    a. *Clinical assessment*: … conduct a thorough clinical assessment, including obtaining a detailed medical history and performing a physical examination. Symptoms may include sudden-onset neurological deficits, such as weakness on one side of the body, difficulty speaking, and altered consciousness.
    b. *Neuroimaging*: Neuroimaging studies, such as magnetic resonance imaging (MRI) or computed tomography (CT) scans, are essential for diagnosing stroke and determining its location and extent.
    c. *Laboratory tests*:
        • *Hemoglobin electrophoresis*: To confirm the presence of SCD and rule out other hemoglobinopathies.
        • *Complete blood count (CBC)*: To assess the degree of anemia and reticulocytosis.
        • *Coagulation studies*: To rule out other causes of stroke, such as clotting disorders.
2. *Management*:
    The management of stroke in individuals with sickle cell disease involves several components, including acute treatment, secondary prevention, and supportive care:
    a. *Acute treatment*:
        • *Blood transfusion*: Exchange transfusion or simple transfusion may be administered to raise hemoglobin levels, decrease the percentage of sickled red blood cells, and improve oxygen delivery to the brain.
        • *Intravenous fluids*: Hydration and adequate blood pressure management are essential to prevent further sickling and improve blood flow.
        • *Neurological assessment*: Frequent neurological assessments are crucial to monitor the patient's condition and response to treatment.
    b. *Secondary prevention*:
        • *Chronic transfusion therapy*: Some individuals at high risk of recurrent stroke may be placed on chronic transfusion therapy to maintain hemoglobin S levels below a certain threshold and prevent further strokes.
        • *Hydroxyurea*: In some cases, hydroxyurea, a medication that increases the production of fetal hemoglobin, may be prescribed to reduce the frequency of vaso-occlusive events.…

- *Supportive care*: Supportive measures, including pain management, management of complications, and psychosocial support, are essential for overall well-being.

Algorithm: see **Chapter 15**

23

Deep Venous Thrombosis (DVT)/Central Venous Thrombosis

Clots may be incidental and asymptomatic and can occur anywhere but most often present with pain, swelling, discoloration, coolness, and decreased pulses due to poor perfusion. Findings usually will be unilateral but can be bilateral as when the common iliac vein is occluded with extension to both iliac veins. CNS clots can be associated with strokes (especially **cerebral sinus venous thrombosis** such as those due to **asparaginase**), seizures, and secondary bleeding due to "back up" pressure. *SVC syndrome* may be a presentation of clots in the neck or mediastinum. Patients with suspected peripheral clots usually will have had peripheral vascular Doppler ultrasounds (PVLs) completed before you are called. PVL reports should be reviewed for which vessel is involved, whether it is a vein or artery, and where possible distal and proximal extent. In many centers these can only be done during the day. Veins may be **superficial (brachiocephalic, saphenous)** or deep (including **any femoral vein involvement**), peripheral, or in the CNS, chest, or abdomen. Management includes:

- History: in addition to symptom review (above), context and predisposing causes are important. Ask about prior clots, trauma in the area of clot, central lines, and other high-risk features— adjacent infection, increased inflammation, obesity, immobility, cancer, burns, cyanotic heart disease, severe dehydration, protein-losing disorder, drugs such as estrogen-containing birth control or asparaginase; family history of clots, heart attacks at an age earlier than "old". *COVID*, more than most viral infections, is a prothrombotic or hypercoagulable state. Keep an eye out for respiratory distress that may signal **pulmonary embolus**;
  - Know about (relative) contraindications to anticoagulation: CNS hemorrhage, other major bleeding or uncorrected coagulopathy, epidural in place or immediate plans for surgery, low platelets ($<50,000/mm^3$);
- Laboratory studies, which may be refined based on history, should include:
  - Baseline CBC diff, PT/INR, and PTT with 1:1 mixing study, D-dimer;
  - Chem screen to inform anticoagulation choices, urinalysis to look for nephrotic syndrome (which leads to loss of clotting and anti-clotting factors in the urine);

- Thrombophilia work-up: Patients without an obvious provoked clot (e.g., central line) should be considered for a thrombophilia work-up, most of which can be done after initiation of antioagulation. However, it may be important to know Anti-Thrombin 3 (AT3) levels as this would affect heparin and lovenox levels. Other work-up includes: protein S and C activity, factor V Leiden (different from plain old factor V levels), and prothrombin (factor II) mutations, and consider an antiphospholipid antibody panel (anticardiolipin IgG and IgM; beta-2 glycoprotein IgG and IgM; lupus anticoagulant); other diagnostic considerations include homocystinuria, SLE, malignancy, homocysteine; think about paroxysmal nocturnal hemoglobinuria (PNH) which can be tested for by flow cytometry;
- COVID testing in this day and age, even without symptoms is not a bad idea (*COVID and Hematologic Emergencies*);
- Imaging in addition to PVLs: Patients with CNS lesions likely will need MRIs or MRAs in addition to uncontrasted CT scans (the latter are good for looking for bleeds). Where clots have intraabdominal or intrathoracic components, CTs may be needed for visualization of the extent of clot. Mechanical compression of the left common iliac vein by the overlying right common iliac artery defines **May–Thurner syndrome** and portal venous or venographic phase CTs may be needed for diagnosis. **Thoracic outlet syndromes** involve compression of veins draining the upper extremities. Talk with your radiology colleagues about the best diagnostic imaging;
- Treatment often needs to proceed without having yet defined an underlying etiology, and is designed to decrease the risks of thrombus progression or recurrence, **pulmonary emboli**, and post-thrombotic syndrome (lymphedema in an involved extremity);
  - VTE that is an incidental finding and has been asymptomatic may not require anticoagulation. If such a patient is seen as a night-time consult, he/she/they may not need to be admitted so long as follow-up can be arranged over the next 1–2 weeks. Offending catheters should be removed if no longer needed;
  - **Superficial clots** (above) often can be managed with supportive care (heat, elevation of involved body part, compression) and **do not always need systemic therapy. However, this can be considered for high-risk patients;**
  - Initial therapy options (almost always as an in-patient to facilitate education and dose adjustments) include:
    - UnFractionated Heparin (UFH) especially for patients with increased bleeding risk or for whom surgical interventions are planned soon, since UFH can be quickly eliminated from the body just by stopping infusions. Most centers have algorithms for adjusting doses and you usually can ask the pharmacy for help. Patients with **cerebral sinus venous thrombosis may need anticoagulation even in the presence of hemorrhage;**

- Low molecular weight heparin (LMWH = enoxaparin): for children ≥2 months, 1 mg/kg subcutaneously every 12 hours or fondaparinux 0.1 mg/kg subcutaneously daily. For children <2 months, 1.5 mg/kg bid of LMWH is a good option (see *Neonatal Hematologic Emergencies*);
- Direct oral thrombin (Xa) inhibitors (DOACs) such as rivaroxiban (Xarelto pills or liquid) are increasingly used in children and maybe even in infants although many centers use heparins for 5–7 days before transitioning. Check dose adjustments for obesity, renal failure;
- Consideration for thrombolysis with systemic or local tissue plasminogen activator (TPA) in patients with life- or limb-threatening thromboembolism. Ask Vascular Interventional Radiology to consult even as you start other options. Absolute contraindications to the use of thrombolytics include recent intracranial hemorrhage or stroke, known cerebrovascular abnormality, and malignant intracranial neoplasm. Relative contraindications include recent major surgery, uncontrolled hypertension, and recent significant bleeding episode;
- Thrombectomy can be considered especially for large intracardiac clots. Consult CT surgery as needed;
- Discussion of inferior vena cava (IVC) filters is not for the middle of the night.

Bibliography

Beyer-Westendorf J. Controversies in venous thromboembolism: to treat or not to treat superficial vein thrombosis. *Hematology Am Soc Hematol Educ Program*. 2017;2017(1):223–230.

Cohen CT, Kirk S, Desai SB, et al. Diagnosis, clinical characteristics, and treatment modalities of adolescent May-Thurner syndrome-associated deep venous thrombosis. *J Pediatr Hematol Oncol*. 2021;43:e346–e350.

Desjardins B, Hanley M, Steigler ML, et al. Appropriateness Criteria® suspected upper extremity deep vein thrombosis. Expert panel on vascular imaging. *J Am Coll Radiol*. 2020;17:S315–S322.

Jaffray J, Young G. Deep vein thrombosis in pediatric patients. *Pediatr Blood Cancer*. 2018;65(3). doi: 10.1002/pbc.26881

Monagle P, Cuello CA, Augustine C, et al. American Society of Hematology 2018 Guidelines for management of venous thromboembolism: treatment of pediatric thromboembolism. *Blood Adv*. 2018;2:3292–3316.

What ChatGPT Says

All true but not much in terms of emergency measures for night calls. We can't remember the last time we used venography and never at night. Many of us use DOACs even as a first-line therapy in young children. Warfarin is much harder to regulate, although it is less expensive so may be attractive in some centers.

1. *Clinical assessment*: … conduct a thorough clinical assessment, including obtaining a detailed medical history and performing a physical examination. Symptoms may include pain, swelling, and redness in the affected limb.

2. *Imaging studies*:
   a. Doppler ultrasound.
   b. Venography: In some cases, venography may be performed to provide a more detailed view of the clot, especially if Doppler ultrasound results are inconclusive.

3. *Laboratory tests*:
   a. Blood tests to assess for any underlying hypercoagulable conditions or clotting disorders that may have contributed to the DVT.

4. *Management*:
   a. *Anticoagulation therapy*: The primary treatment for DVT in children is anticoagulation therapy, which involves medications to prevent further clot formation and reduce the risk of complications. Common anticoagulants used in children include low molecular weight heparin (LMWH) and warfarin. The choice of anticoagulant and dosing is individualized based on the child's age, weight, and underlying condition.
   b. *Duration of anticoagulation*: The duration of anticoagulation therapy depends on various factors, including the cause of the DVT and the risk of recurrence. A pediatric hematologist should be consulted to help determine the appropriate treatment duration.
   c. *Monitoring*: Children receiving anticoagulation therapy need regular monitoring of their blood clotting levels to ensure that they are within a therapeutic range and to adjust the medication as needed.
   d. *Compression therapy*: The use of compression stockings or bandages may be recommended to alleviate swelling and discomfort in the affected limb.
   e. *Treatment of underlying conditions*: If an underlying cause of DVT is identified (e.g., a clotting disorder), treatment for that condition may be necessary.

Algorithm: **Deep Venous Thrombosis (DVT)/Central Venous Thrombosis**

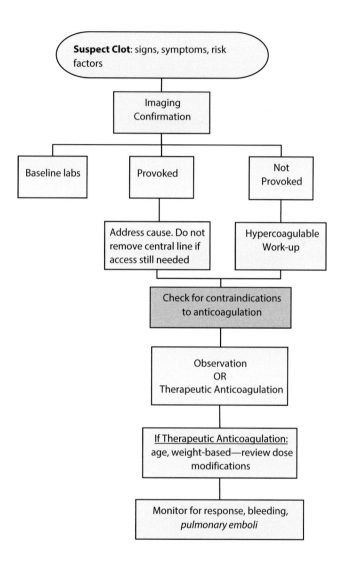

24

Pulmonary Embolus (PE)

Pulmonary embolus (PE) presents as shortness of breath, pleuritic chest pain, cough, dyspnea, or tachycardia often with hypoxia. Approximately 50% of patients will have a concurrent lower extremity *DVT* and most of the laboratory evaluation is the same as for *DVTs*. In some people, PE is present before a known DVT. PE is a **medical emergency** and diagnosis requires:

- Spiral or thin-cut CT or MR angiography;
- If no prior known DVT, order PVL (Peripheral Vascular Laboratory) screen of lower extremities (this can be done a bit more electively);
- Stat echocardiogram (EKG) to look for right ventricular strain which will increase urgency of the work-up;
- Consider tissue plasminogen activator (TPA) and/or thrombectomy for patients with evidence of cardiac compromise (consult vascular interventional radiology and/or CT surgery).

Further evaluation for underlying causes and treatment are essentially the same as for *DVT*. Supplemental O_2 may be needed to maintain saturations >92%.

Bibliography

see Chapter 23

What ChatGPT Says

Same as for *DVT* with the addition of consideration of additional radiographic studies, which we might disagree with.

DOI: 10.1201/9781003473701-26

1. *Imaging studies*:
    a. *Computed Tomography Pulmonary Angiography (CTPA)*: This is the most commonly used imaging study to diagnose PE in both adults and children. It provides detailed images of the pulmonary arteries and can identify the presence of blood clots.
    b. *Ventilation/Perfusion (V/Q) Scanning*: In some cases, when CTPA is contraindicated or unavailable, V/Q scans may be performed to assess lung function and evaluate for areas of reduced perfusion.

Algorithm: **Pulmonary Embolus (PE)**

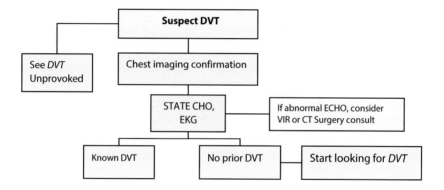

25

Arterial Thrombosis

Arterial thrombosis presents pretty much the same as *DVT* but arterial catheters (notably umbilical artery lines in newborns) and cardiac catheterizations are usual provoking events. Uncorrected congenital cardiac lesions may be set-ups for arterial emboli. So:

- Order Doppler ultrasound for documentation. Almost always arterial thrombi are managed in a PICU or NICU;
- Ask nursing, cardiology, or surgery or interventional radiology (whoever placed the line) to remove the responsible arterial catheter;
- Serial physical exam looking for changes in pain, swelling, discoloration, coolness, and decreased pulses due to poor perfusion;
- For patients with a symptomatic arterial clot, most of us recommend UFH or LMWH until resolution of symptoms or for at least a 7-day trial. Ongoing management is a good discussion for morning rounds;
- Can consider aspirin (dose) +/– other anticoagulants but this discussion also can wait until morning;
- For severe arterial thrombus (life- or limb-threatening) consult IR and CT/vascular surgery for thrombolysis or thrombectomy. Don't be surprised if they defer intervention to see what heparin does;
- Order next-day repeat Doppler US to assess for improvement in blood flow.

What ChatGPT Says

The same as with *DVT* but with a few additions, including recommendations more common in adult medicine and not for nights:

1. *Diagnosis*:
    a. *Imaging studies*:
        - *Doppler ultrasound*: Doppler ultrasound is commonly used to diagnose arterial thrombosis, especially in the extremities.

DOI: 10.1201/9781003473701-27

- *Magnetic Resonance Angiography (MRA) or computed tomography angiography (CTA)*: These imaging studies provide a more detailed view of the affected arteries, helping to identify the location and extent of thrombosis.

b. *Laboratory tests*:

- Blood tests, including a complete blood count (CBC), coagulation studies, and specific clotting disorder tests, may be conducted to assess for underlying conditions or risk factors contributing to arterial thrombosis.

2. *Management*:

The management of arterial thrombosis in childhood involves several components, including treatment to dissolve or remove the clot, prevention of recurrence, and supportive care:

a. *Thrombolytic therapy*: In some cases, thrombolytic therapy with medications like tissue plasminogen activator (tPA) may be considered to dissolve the clot. This treatment is typically used for acute, life-threatening situations such as arterial thrombosis involving the brain, heart, or other vital organs.

b. *Anticoagulation therapy*: After an arterial thrombosis event, anticoagulation therapy is initiated to prevent further clot formation and reduce the risk of complications. The choice of anticoagulant and dosing is individualized based on the child's age, weight, and underlying condition.

c. *Interventional procedures*: In some cases, interventional procedures, such as angioplasty and stent placement, may be necessary to mechanically remove or open up the clot.

d. *Treatment of underlying conditions*: Identification and management of underlying conditions contributing to arterial thrombosis, such as clotting disorders, are important to prevent recurrences.

e. *Supportive care*: Depending on the location and severity of the thrombosis, supportive care may be needed. This may include pain management, monitoring for organ dysfunction, and measures to stabilize the patient's condition.

Algorithm: **Arterial Thrombosis**

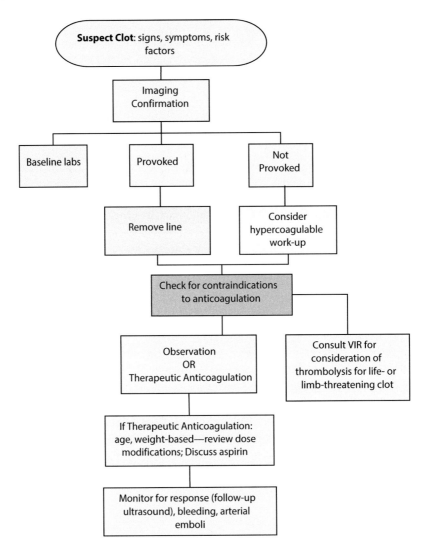

26

Arterial (Acute Ischemic) Stroke

Arterial (acute ischemic) stroke is a rare event in pediatrics, occurs most commonly in the newborn period, and *SCD* is the most commonly associated hematologic disorder outside of that age group. Other predisposing conditions include cardiac disease, recent cardiac catheterization, and hypertension. Acute ischemic strokes are rarely associated with inherited thrombophilias. Ischemia must be distinguished from hemorrhage which also can cause strokes. Neonates with strokes may present with lethargy, seizures, or coma while older children also can have acute focal neurologic changes. Emergency management includes:

- Stat neurology and PICU consults even before documentation with imaging. **These are usually the people who primarily manage strokes**, although you may be asked for input overnight;
- Imaging, ideally brain MRI/MRA. Screening with an uncontrasted brain CT is quicker and can rule out hemorrhage but may miss small lesions and acute events (<12–24 hours old);
- EKG and echocardiogram should be obtained in all children with strokes to assess for a possible cardioembolic source;
- Neuroprotective measures—fever reduction, seizure control, maintaining normoglycemia, and avoiding hypotension when treating hypertension. There remains controversy regarding the use of anti-platelet agents (usually aspirin to start) vs anticoagulation therapy in pediatric patients. However, some centers anticoagulate neonates with strokes even in the presence of associated hemorrhage;
- Labs: AT3, homocysteine, factor 5 Leiden and factor 2 mutations, protein C and S levels, and consider maternal APLA.

Bibliography

Ferriero DM, Fullerton HJ, Bernard TJ, et al. Management of stroke in neonates and children: A scientific statement from the American Heart Association/American Stroke Association. *Stroke.* 2019;50:e51–e96.

Sporns PB, Fullerton HJ, Lee S, et al. Current treatment for childhood arterial ischaemic stroke. *Lancet Child Adolesc Health.* 2021;5:825–836.

DOI: 10.1201/9781003473701-28

What ChatGPT Says

Way too vague:

1. *Diagnosis*:
   a. *Clinical assessment* … detailed medical history and performing a physical examination. Symptoms may include sudden-onset neurological deficits, such as weakness on one side of the body, difficulty speaking, and altered consciousness.
   b. *Imaging studies*:
      - *Magnetic resonance imaging (MRI)*: MRI is the preferred imaging modality for diagnosing ischemic stroke in children. It provides detailed images of the brain and helps identify the location and extent of the stroke.
      - *Computed tomography (CT) Scan*: In some cases, a CT scan may be used if MRI is unavailable or contraindicated. It can quickly identify large, acute strokes.
   c. *Vascular imaging*: Depending on the clinical presentation and age of the child, vascular imaging studies such as magnetic resonance angiography (MRA) or computed tomography angiography (CTA) may be performed to assess blood vessels and identify underlying causes.
   d. *Blood tests*: Blood tests may be conducted to evaluate for underlying conditions or risk factors contributing to the stroke. This includes coagulation studies and clotting disorder tests.
2. *Management*:
   a. *Acute treatment*:
      - *Thrombolytic therapy*: In some cases, thrombolytic therapy with medications like tissue plasminogen activator (tPA) may be considered, but it is less common in children compared to adults. Thrombolytic therapy is typically used in select cases when the benefits outweigh the risks, and it must be administered within a strict time window.
      - *Anticoagulation or antiplatelet therapy*: Anticoagulants or antiplatelet medications may be considered to prevent further clot formation and reduce the risk of complications. The choice of medication and dosing is individualized based on the child's age, weight, and underlying condition.
   b. *Prevention of complications*: Monitoring and management of complications such as seizures, infections, or recurrent strokes is essential.

Algorithm

If you know how to pick up a telephone and reach PICU and Neurology, you will NOT need an algorithm. What you don't do is almost as important as what you do do—most of us do not embark on a major hypercoagulation work-up and if we do, this can wait until the morning.

27

Heparin Induced Thrombocytopenia (HIT)

Heparin induced thrombocytopenia (HIT) is not that common in pediatrics but can occur and be a cause of thrombosis/stroke requiring urgent attention. Most patients will have been receiving anticoagulation with heparins (UFH or LMWH) but HIT can occur even when heparin exposure is limited to KVO treatment of peripheral intravenous lines (PIVs). Rarer still is **spontaneous HIT** in someone who has never been exposed to heparins, usually in the setting of autoimmune disease or viral infection. Monitoring for HIT (not your problem on nights) has been risk-stratified using the **4Ts score** (see Hwang 2005–2024) and ranges from no monitoring for low-risk patients to daily CBCs (see references for timing). Suspect HIT when the baseline platelet count drops by 20% or more, even if not low, and especially **when a patient has new or progressive thrombosis while on anticoagulation**. Immediate management will depend on 4T risk but for intermediate or high-risk patients (4T ≥ 3) includes:

- Stopping all use of heparins including in PIV lines;
- Substitute argatroban (0.75 mcg/kg/minute continuous IV infusion), bivalrudin (Angiomax, Angioox 0.3 mcg/kg/hr continuous IV infusion) or fondaparinox (Arixtra 0.1 mg/kg/dose subq once daily);
- Send HIT panel (immunoassay). This may not result overnight so **don't** wait for this to intervene, but **do** check results on days;
- Once HIT is confirmed, document in chart and **do not** rechallenge.

Bibliography

Avila ML, Shah V, Brandão LR. Systematic review on heparin-induced thrombocytopenia in children: a call to action. *J Thromb Haemost*. 2013;11:660–669.

Becker CJ, Heston AL, Carrera JF. Spontaneous heparin-induced thrombocytopenia presenting as acute ischemic stroke. *Neurol Clin Pract*. 2021;11:e918–e920.

Cuker A, Arepally GM, Chong BH, et al. American Society of Hematology 2018 Guidelines for management of venous thromboembolism: heparin-induced thrombocytopenia. *Blood Adv*. 2018; 2:3360–3392.

Hwang C. 4Ts score for heparin-induced thrombocytopenia, MDCalc, 2005–2024, available at: https://www.mdcalc.com/calc/1787/4ts-score-heparin-induced-thrombocytopenia

What ChatGPT Says

Not bad! Especially for the non-hematologist pediatricians seeing these patients:

1. *Clinical assessment*: ... clinical assessment, including obtaining a detailed medical history and performing a physical examination. Symptoms may include a decrease in platelet count, unexplained thrombosis (blood clots), and other signs of clot-related complications.

2. *Laboratory tests*:

   a. *Platelet count*: A significant decrease in platelet count (usually >50% drop from baseline) is a hallmark of HIT.

   b. *HIT antibody testing*: HIT is an immune-mediated disorder, and specific blood tests, such as enzyme-linked immunosorbent assay (ELISA) and serotonin release assay (SRA), can be performed to detect antibodies to heparin-platelet factor 4 complexes.

3. *Management*:

   The management of heparin-induced thrombocytopenia in childhood involves several components, including the immediate discontinuation of heparin, treatment of thrombosis, and alternative anticoagulation strategies:

   a. *Immediate discontinuation of heparin*: The first step is to discontinue all heparin products, including unfractionated heparin and low molecular weight heparin (LMWH).

      - *Treatment of thrombosis*:
        - If thrombosis is present, children may require treatment with alternative anticoagulants, such as direct thrombin inhibitors (e.g., argatroban, bivalirudin) or fondaparinux, to prevent further clot formation.
        - In some cases, children may need thrombectomy or other interventional procedures to manage thrombosis, especially if it is causing severe complications.

   b. *Platelet transfusions*: Platelet transfusions are generally avoided in HIT, as they can exacerbate the thrombotic risk and may be ineffective. The management focus is on anticoagulation to prevent and treat thrombosis.

   c. *Consultation with specialists*: Collaboration with hematologists and other specialists experienced in the care of patients with HIT is essential for managing this condition in children.

   d. *Use of non-heparin anticoagulants*: For anticoagulation needs, alternative agents that do not cross-react with HIT antibodies may be used. This may include the use of direct oral anticoagulants (DOACs) like apixaban or rivaroxaban, warfarin, or other agents based on the specific clinical situation.

   e. *Monitoring*: Regular monitoring of platelet counts and assessment of thrombotic risk are important to guide ongoing treatment and anticoagulation strategies.

   f. *Prevention*: In children with a history of HIT, the use of heparin should be avoided in the future, and an alternative anticoagulant should be used if necessary.

Algorithm: **Heparin Induced Thrombocytopenia (HIT)**

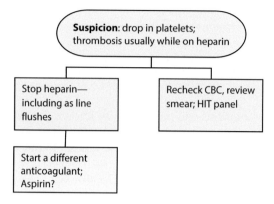

28

Bleeding Emergencies

These can occur in two situations—in patients with known predisposing conditions or in patients presenting for the first time with serious bleeding. The first setting, in an inpatient or with an ER visit and a call to you as the on-call hematologist, about management and possible need for admission is usually straightforward (see *Thrombocytopenia, Hemophilia, VWD, Vitamin K Deficiency*, and *Other Factor Deficiencies*). The second situation takes a bit more thought. Newborns are a different species, at least lab-wise, so see *Neonatal Hematologic Emergencies*. For everyone else:

- Stat lab tests should probably be sent off even before a more detailed history:
  - CBC diff and look at peripheral blood smear later for platelet clumping or RBC microangiopathy (schistocytes). You can ask the lab to look at peripheral smear as well, but this may be something **you** will need to do also overnight (see *Thrombotic Microangiopathy*);
  - PT/INR, PTT with a 1:1 mixing study if screens are elevated (normalization confirms factor deficiency, lack of normalization suggests an inhibitor—usually not a reason for bleeding);
  - CMP to look for renal disease (acquired platelet dysfunction is not usually seen except in end-stage renal disease), liver disease (coagulopathy due to poor synthetic function);
  - Isolated elevated PT/INR: Most frequently from early *Vitamin K Deficiency* although later stages would also have high PTT due to factor 2, 9, or 10 deficiency; can be early liver disease as well or the rare congenital factor 7 deficiency;

    Isolated elevated aPTT: Factors 8, 9, 11, or 12 deficiency (12 deficiency is **almost** never a reason for bleeding), heparin contamination, lupus anticoagulant, or severe *VWD*. Stat factor 8 and 9, especially in boys, are needed in the face of severe bleeding, even with no family history. This may require the transfer of a child to your tertiary care center if an outside hospital can't do it;
  - Consider Factor 13 if INR and PTT are normal or if Factor 12 deficiency is the only abnormality, particularly in the setting of intracranial hemorrhage;
  - Grab a type & cross and keep an IV in place until you know if infusions/transfusions are needed;
  - Urinalysis or urine dip to look for blood (red cells, not just Hgb) since hematuria is a contraindication to antifibrinolytics;
  - Imaging such as a non-contrast CT scan to look for bleeding may be indicated emergently but not until after a patient has been appropriately stabilized (e.g.,

DOI: 10.1201/9781003473701-30

platelet transfusions for suspected major bleeding due to low platelets, factor infusions in hemophiliacs).

- History will go a long way to determining the reason for bleeding and may result in the addition of more labs.
  - Unusual bruising, petechiae, mucocutaneous bleeding (bilateral epistaxis/gingival bleeding), prolonged bleeding after surgery or dental extractions, hematuria or gastrointestinal bleeding (black or bright red stools), or heavy menstrual bleeding suggest a problem with platelets, Von Willebrand factor, and/or vasculature (e.g., the rare Ehlers-Danlos type 3);
  - Soft tissue, muscle, or joint bleeds, delayed bleeding with lacerations or following surgery (including circumcision), and patients with spontaneous intracranial hemorrhages are more likely to be the result of a defect in the coagulation cascade (*Hemophilia, Other Factor Deficiencies*). The distinctions are not absolute and some patients with coagulation defects may have mucocutaneous bleeding;
  - Some abnormalities are inherited and family history is helpful if a knowledgeable family member is available. So is knowing whether a patient is a boy or girl—which should be apparent after history and physical exam;
  - Does the patient have signs and symptoms of infection which can cause consumptive coagulopathy. Although disseminated intravascular coagulation (DIC) most commonly results from sepsis, it can also be caused by trauma, APML, certain vascular anomalies. Diagnostic studies include thrombocytopenia, low fibrinogen, elevated D-Dimer from ongoing fibrinolysis, elevated PT/PTT, and schistocytes on peripheral blood smear. In cases where factor levels are measured a low factor V and factor VIII will distinguish DIC from failure of hepatic synthesis in which factor 8 levels are preserved. Ask about medications—some, like ibuprofen, screw up platelet function; others, like antibiotics, can cause *vitamin K deficiency*. Get the history and worry about what meds do what later;
  - Changes in mental status, seizures, motor function, or other neurologic abnormalities will need to speed up the work-up but by then you probably will have called a rapid response and gotten some help, maybe with a transfer to the PICU;
- A detailed physical exam after a cursory look for where the bleeding is and a set of VS with a weight to help with dosing should follow. Neurologic status (abnormal with CNS or spinal/paraspinal bleeds; see *Spinal/Paraspinal Mass* and *Thrombotic Microangiopathy (TMA)*;
- It is worth noting that you may get consulted on nights about a suspected non-accidental trauma (NAT). While this is not usually a PHO emergency, you would feel pretty dumb if it was determined that the child did have a hematologic reason for or compounding bleeding. Consider treating these as emergencies and at least order the labs just mentioned.

By this point, if the child is not already transferred for more acute care, you probably have a pretty good idea as to the diagnosis. However, a few comments about interventions are worth considering, regardless of the etiology for the bleeding:

- If transfusions are needed, recheck Hgb levels at least 4 hours after (to allow equilibration);

- Treatment of mucocutaneous bleeding begins with local measures including pressure, topical therapy (topical thrombin/fibrin sealant), and antifibrinolytics (amicar [50 mg/kg q6hr IV or PO with a max dose of 5 g q6hr] or tranexamic acid [Lysteda 20–40 mg/kg/d div bid or tid max dose of 1,300 mg q8hr PO]) will get you started).

Bibliography

See *Thrombocytopenia with/without Bleeding* and *Hemophilia*, Chapter 29

What ChatGPT Says

Not granular enough to help. Maybe a good overview.

The diagnosis and management of these emergencies depend on the specific situation and underlying cause. Here are the key steps in diagnosing and managing bleeding emergencies in childhood:

1. *Diagnosis*:
   a. *Clinical assessment*… conduct a thorough clinical assessment, including obtaining a detailed medical history and performing a physical examination. Symptoms may include uncontrolled bleeding, excessive bruising, or other signs of hemorrhage.
   b. *Laboratory tests*:
      - Complete Blood Count (CBC)
      - *Coagulation studies*: prothrombin time (PT), activated partial thromboplastin time (aPTT), and international normalized ratio (INR) …
      - *Specific clotting disorder tests*: Depending on the clinical presentation, specific tests for clotting disorders may be necessary to identify any underlying conditions, such as hemophilia or von Willebrand disease.
2. *Management*:
   The management of bleeding emergencies in childhood varies based on the severity of bleeding, the underlying cause, and the specific situation. Here are some general principles for managing bleeding emergencies in children:
   a. *Control bleeding*: The immediate priority is to control active bleeding. This can be achieved through direct pressure on the bleeding site, elevation of the affected limb, and the use of pressure bandages or tourniquets when necessary.
   b. *Fluid resuscitation*: If a child has lost a significant amount of blood, they may require fluid resuscitation to maintain blood pressure and circulation. Intravenous (IV) fluids may be administered in the hospital setting.

c. *Blood transfusions*: Children with severe bleeding and low hemoglobin levels may require blood transfusions, including packed red blood cells or platelets, to replace lost blood components.

d. *Clotting factor replacement*: In cases of bleeding due to clotting disorders, the administration of specific clotting factors or products (e.g., factor VIII or IX for hemophilia) may be necessary to achieve hemostasis.

e. *Medication management*: In some bleeding emergencies, medications to promote clotting or to control bleeding (e.g., tranexamic acid) may be used.

f. *Treatment of underlying causes*: In cases of clotting disorders, addressing the underlying condition is essential. This may involve long-term management with prophylactic clotting factor replacement, medications, and lifestyle modifications.

g. *Surgical intervention*: In certain situations, surgical interventions may be required to address the cause of bleeding or to stop severe hemorrhage.

Algorithm: **Bleeding Emergencies**

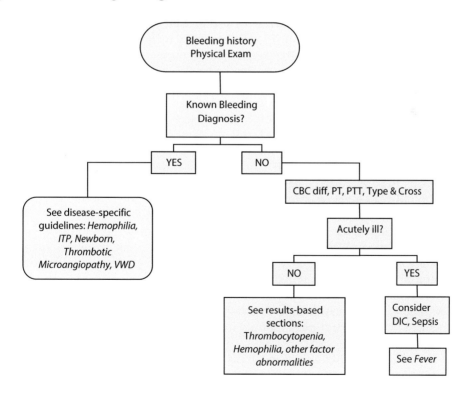

29

Thrombocytopenia With/Without Bleeding

Thrombocytopenia (platelet count <150,000/mm³ except in a newborn where normal levels can be as low as 80–100,000/mm³) is usually not a night-time emergency unless the counts are very low—enough to pose a bleeding risk—or if the context suggests a life-threatening problem such as leukemia (*High White Blood Cell Count*), TMA (*Thrombotic Microangiopathy*), HIT. Patients presenting with symptomatic bleeding associated with thrombocytopenia, whether cutaneous (petechiae and/or ecchymoses), mucosal ("wet purpura"), or severe/life-threatening bleeds (GI, urinary tract, CNS, pulmonary) generally present to urgent care or to the ER. Emergency interventions typically won't start with you on the inpatient service. Such bleeding is unusual unless the platelet count is <20,000/mm³ or 50,000/mm³ in the face of trauma. The clinical history and physical exam will guide your work-up and recommendations. The etiology of thrombocytopenia can be broken down into four simple categories: **failure of production** can be due to infection, cancer, bone marrow failure syndromes, nutritional deficiency including iron deficiency, or drug toxicity. Viral infections are easily the most common reason for the failure of production; **increased destruction** (immune thrombocytopenia [ITP]; *sequestration* or organomegaly); other **increased consumption** as with hemorrhage, or **type 2B VW** in which platelets bind high-molecular-weight VWF, resulting in their increased clearance; and rarely **dilutional**, as seen with massive transfusions in the OR. Emergency interventions (transfusion, drugs) will depend on symptoms and suspected etiology. Although bone marrow evaluation with aspirates or biopsies may be indicated in patients with suspected cancer, almost never is this a middle-of-the-night decision. If you are being called from the ER to ask whether the child needs to be admitted, health-related quality of life concerns are very important (patient age, fall risk, level of education/understanding, socio-economic status, reliable follow-up including telephone access). Some patients can be returned to your colleagues in the outpatient clinic later in the week. However, sometimes in the middle of the night it is just easier to admit and talk more the next day. Before we forget, **thrombocytosis** also is almost never a night-time emergency, and in children **clotting is rare with platelet counts <2 million/mm³**. With counts that high in a well patient, consider admission for dilutional IV fluids and regroup in the AM. If a patient has neurologic symptoms, that is a time to call your attending. No more on this topic for now!

Management of thrombocytopenia should include:

- Review of CBC and differential, mean platelet volume (MPV), and ideally a look at the peripheral blood smear to be sure there is no platelet clumping with a falsely low platelet count, and that the lab isn't missing blasts. High MPV suggests platelet destruction/consumption. Small platelets are uncommon but can be seen in

DOI: 10.1201/9781003473701-31

Wiskott-Aldrich Syndrome. In the middle of the night, one might argue that the fellow would be forgiven if he/she/they called the lab and asked the tech to look for these things; if you have urgent/emergent concerns that will affect treatment decisions, the on-call pathologist may be able to review slides remotely;

- If ITP is in the differential (and it is both one of the only things that causes an isolated severe thrombocytopenia and one of the more common reasons for a middle-of-the-night admission for low platelets), consider a red cell antibody screen and DAT (direct antibody or Coombs test), and an anti-nuclear antibody (ANA) test. A positive red cell antibody screen by inference suggests that anti-platelet antibodies also are present (these are a whole lot harder to test for) and provide a diagnosis of Evans syndrome (autoimmune *hemolytic anemia* with thrombocytopenia). **Patients with Evans syndrome don't have to be anemic or hemolyzing**, and also may have autoimmune neutropenia (sometimes an anti-neutrophil antibody test, not to be confused with an ANA, can be helpful). ITP patients can be anemic from bleeding even if they don't have Evans syndrome, so not all patients with ITP and anemia have Evans syndrome. Antibody screens usually are ordered as part of a type & screen. This may be helpful if you anticipate bleeding and a need for red cell transfusions;

- Depending on the presentation, clinical history and exam findings, consider CMP, uric acid, phosphorous, and LDH (a normal level makes hemolysis and malignancy less likely although still possible);

- In infants less than 1 year of age and adolescent patients with isolated thrombocytopenia, acute ITP is less common, and additional testing for a predisposing immunologic disorder such as HIV or syphilis, should be considered;

- Serial observation for bleeding; apply pressure to blood draw sites;

- While awaiting labs, back to history and physical exam—ITP most commonly occurs in children 2–10 years of age, often with an antecedent viral infection (though this is so common as to be laughable as a diagnostic criterion). Patients typically won't have adenopathy or organomegaly though they might if still in the throes of active infection;

- **Not every very low platelet count in the absence of bleeding needs to be treated** and certainly not emergently but if the decision is made to give a platelet transfusion, a **1- and 24-hour post-platelet transfusion platelet count** can help you to differentiate etiology;
  - Failure of production: Appropriate platelet increase at hour 1 AND sustained at hour 24; increased non-immune destruction or consumption: appropriate platelet increase at hour 1 BUT not sustained at hour 24; immune-mediated: no significant early or late platelet increase;

- If ITP is the best clinical diagnosis, options are suggested below. Anti-D comes with a Black Box warning as it can cause life-threatening *hemolytic anemia*, and we do not use this at our institution. Promacta can be considered first-line therapy for ITP but is rarely initiated emergently;

- Keep less common reasons for low platelets, such as *VW Type 2*, in the back of your mind.

Bibliography

Bussel JB. Immune thrombocytopenia in children: initial management. Post TW, ed. UpToDate. Waltham, MA: UpToDate Inc. http://www.uptodate.com. (Accessed June 8, 2023).

Neunert C. Approach to the child with unexplained thrombocytopenia. Post TW, ed. UpToDate. Waltham, MA: UpToDate Inc. http://www.uptodate.com. (Accessed June 8, 2023).

Sahi PK, Chandra J. Immune thrombocytopenia: American Society of Hematology Guidelines, 2019. *Indian Pediatr*. 2020;57:854–856.

Schifferli A, Holbro A, Chitlur M, Coslovsky M. et al. Intercontinental Cooperative ITP Study Group (ICIS). A comparative prospective observational study of children and adults with immune thrombocytopenia: 2-year follow-up. *Am J Hematol*. 2018;93:751–759.

Tyrrell L, Scruggs M, Kerwin A, Kahwash SB. The role of peripheral blood smear examination in the evaluation of suspected platelet-related disorders in children: a practical approach and an illustrated review. *Malays J Pathol*. 2022;44:397–413.

What ChatGPT Says

Too vague to be helpful:

1. *Clinical assessment*: … conduct a thorough clinical assessment, including obtaining a detailed medical history and performing a physical examination. Symptoms may include easy bruising, nosebleeds, gum bleeding, and, in severe cases, spontaneous bleeding.

2. *Laboratory tests*:

    a. *Complete Blood Count (CBC)*: This test measures platelet counts and assesses other blood cell components. Thrombocytopenia is defined as a platelet count below the reference range for a child's age.

    b. *Peripheral blood smear*: This test allows for the examination of blood cells under a microscope and can help identify any structural abnormalities in platelets.

    c. *Bone marrow aspiration and biopsy*: In some cases, a bone marrow examination may be performed to determine the underlying cause of thrombocytopenia, especially if other diagnostic tests do not yield a clear diagnosis.

3. *Evaluation for underlying causes*: Depending on the clinical presentation and initial test results, further investigations may be needed to identify any underlying conditions contributing to thrombocytopenia. These can include:

    a. Viral infections (e.g., Epstein–Barr virus)

    b. Medication-induced thrombocytopenia

    c. Immune thrombocytopenic purpura (ITP)

    d. Inherited platelet disorders

   e. Leukemia

   f. Autoimmune disorders

   g. Other bone marrow disorders

4. *Management*:

The management of thrombocytopenia in childhood is highly dependent on the underlying cause and the severity of the condition:

   a. *Management of underlying conditions*:

   - If thrombocytopenia is caused by an underlying condition, such as a viral infection or medication, addressing the root cause is the primary approach. Discontinuing the medication or treating the infection may resolve the thrombocytopenia.

   - In cases of leukemia or other bone marrow disorders, specialized treatment and consultation with pediatric hematologists/oncologists are necessary.

   b. *Immune thrombocytopenic purpura (ITP)*:

   - In cases of ITP, which is an autoimmune condition, the management approach may include observation without treatment in mild cases.

   - In more severe cases of ITP, treatment options may include corticosteroids, intravenous immunoglobulin (IVIG), and anti-D immunoglobulin.

   - In refractory or chronic ITP, additional treatments, such as thrombopoietin receptor agonists or splenectomy, may be considered.

   c. *Platelet transfusions*: Platelet transfusions may be considered in cases of severe thrombocytopenia with active bleeding or prior to invasive procedures that carry a risk of bleeding.

   - *Identify the cause*: Thrombocytopenia can have various underlying causes, such as immune-mediated disorders, infections, medication side effects, or bone marrow disorders. It's important to identify and address the specific cause to guide further management.

   - *Monitor and manage bleeding*: Close monitoring of the patient's bleeding symptoms and response to treatment is essential. Depending on the severity of bleeding, additional interventions such as surgical measures or specific medications may be required to control bleeding effectively.

Algorithm: Thrombocytopenia With or Without Bleeding

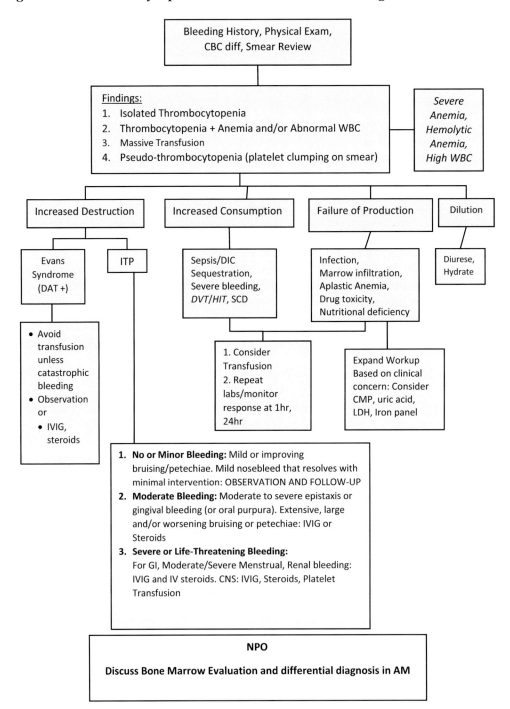

30

Hemophilia

Hemophilia A (Factor VIII deficiency) and B (Factor IX deficiency) are X-linked deficiencies and occur mostly but not only in males. **Female carriers can be as symptomatic as patients with mild hemophilia.** Hemophilia C (Factor XI deficiency, see *Other Factor Deficiencies*) is an autosomal recessive with equal opportunity for males and females. Although family histories often are positive on the mother's side, hemophilia can also be caused by de novo mutations in patients with no relevant family history. The severity of illness is determined by the level of clotting factor activity (<1% of normal is considered severe; 1–5% moderate; 6–50% mild) which you will know after having done the evaluation suggested in the section *Bleeding Emergencies*. Most spontaneous emergencies (i.e., other than those due to trauma) will be in patients with severe disease and life-threatening locations including the brain, spine, airway, iliopsoas area, retroperitoneum, and GI tract. For patients with known hemophilia who present with bleeding, management includes:

- **Treat first, ask questions later!** Empiric factor dosing with factor **before a patient leaves the ER/floor for confirmatory imaging studies.** Ideally, target a factor level of 80–100 IU/dL for life-threatening emergencies. **Clinic notes and families should indicate what factor product a patient has gotten** and should get. In general, 1 unit/kg of factor 8 will raise the level by 2% (50 u/kg should get you to 100%). 1 unit/kg of factor 9 will raise the level by only 1%. For previously untreated patients, see what replacement factors are in your institutional formulary. In patients with suspected hemophilia **before documentation of specific factor deficiency** (e.g., based on prolonged PTT alone), **unless there is a good family history, do not treat with targeted factor replacement** (send blood for testing and consider (partially) correcting PTT as needed with FFP until results available);

- Early recognition of an iliopsoas bleed in hemophilia patients is essential as patients can lose a large amount of blood leading to *severe anemia* or intra-abdominal compartment syndrome:
  - Symptoms include pain in the hip, groin, lower abdomen, or buttock; pain with ambulation, hip held in flexion, numbness and tingling in the leg. May mimic appendicitis;

- Although factor levels after treatment can help assess for the presence of an inhibitor, this is not usually a middle-of-the-night consideration;

- Nonetheless, suspect an inhibitor when patients don't respond as anticipated based on post-treatment factor levels or lack of clinical improvement. "Bypassing agents," such as an activated prothrombin complex concentrate (aPCC) (i.e. Feiba [50–100 u/kg q 12 hours] or novo-7 [90 mcg/kg q 2–3 hours]), can be given to patients with known inhibitors. While special tests can confirm the presence of inhibitors, these same agents can be given emergently even before an inhibitor is documented. Novo 7 can be ordered for 2–3 doses with re-evaluation for efficacy;

- **FEIBA should not be used with antifibrinolytics or given to patients already on Emicizumab** (Hemlibra), a newly approved monoclonal antibody that is given subcutaneously and is used as prophylaxis to prevent bleeding in patients with hemophilia A with or without inhibitors. The combination can promote thrombosis.

___

Bibliography

Matuk-Villazon O, Roberts JC, Corrales-Medina FF. Hemophilia: The past, the present, the future. *Pediatr Rev.* 2021;42:672–683.

Robertson JD, Curtin JA, Blanchdette VS. Managing Hemophilia in children and adolescents, in: Blanchette VS, Brandão LR, Brekey VR, Revel-Vilk S, eds, *SickKids Handbook of Pediatric Thrombosis and Hemostasis*. 2nd ed. Karger 2017.

World Federation of Hemophilia. *Guidelines for the Management of Hemophilia*. 2nd ed.; originally published in Haemophilia 2012. Available at: https://hemophilia.weill.cornell.edu/sites/default/files/whf_guidelines.pdf

___

What ChatGPT Says

We share the most relevant responses regarding emergency care to "How to treat hemophilia." Not much granularity:

1. *Management*:

    The management of hemophilia in childhood aims to prevent bleeding episodes and treat any bleeding that occurs. It typically involves a multidisciplinary approach and includes the following components:

    a. *Clotting factor replacement therapy*:

       - Children with hemophilia receive clotting factor replacement therapy to increase the levels of the missing or deficient clotting factor in their blood. This can be administered as prophylaxis (regularly scheduled infusions) or on-demand (in response to bleeding).

       - Hemophilia A is treated with factor VIII replacement, and hemophilia B is treated with factor IX replacement.

    b. *Prophylactic treatment*: Prophylactic treatment is the administration of clotting factor concentrates on a regular schedule to prevent bleeding episodes. This is the standard of care for severe hemophilia and aims to maintain factor levels within a target range.

    c. *On-demand treatment*: On-demand treatment involves administering clotting factor concentrates when a bleeding episode occurs. Prompt treatment is essential to prevent complications.

d. *Home infusion*: Some families are trained to perform home infusions, which can help improve the child's quality of life by reducing the need for frequent hospital visits.

e. *Management of bleeding episodes*: If a bleeding episode occurs, it is important to treat it promptly with the appropriate factor replacement. This may require adjusting the dose based on the severity of the bleed.

f. *Joint care*: Children with hemophilia, particularly severe forms, are at risk of bleeding into joints, which can lead to joint damage over time. Regular physical therapy and joint protection strategies are important to maintain joint health.

g. *Pain management*: Pain associated with bleeding episodes should be managed with pain relievers and, in some cases, joint aspirations and other joint interventions.

Algorithm: **Hemophilia**

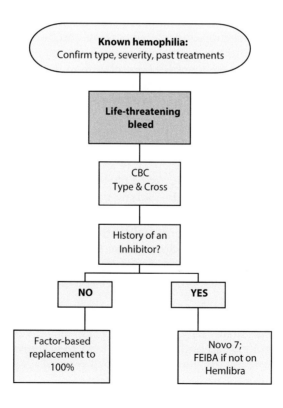

31

Von Willebrand Disease (VWD)

Von Willebrand Disease (VWD) clinically is a bit of a hybrid and can present similar to a platelet problem with epistaxis, gingival bleeding, heavy menstrual bleeding, or as a coagulation factor deficiency with hemarthrosis. This is not the place to review the many types of VWD (types 1, 2A, 2B, 2M, 2N, 3), but 75% of patients will have type 1 VWD which is usually mild and doesn't often come up as a night-time emergency. Intracranial hemorrhage is extremely rare. Suspicion of VWD, raised by the patient's history and family history, requires confirmation with a screening VW "panel" that includes VWF activity, VWF antigen levels, and factor 8 levels. Repeat testing over 6 months is technically required for confirmation of diagnosis unless genetic testing is done. However, that is an issue for your outpatient hemophilia team. It is worth checking a blood type, since people with Type O have lower normative levels of VW activity and antigen than do the rest of the population. As noted in the prior section, low platelet counts can be seen in patients with type 2B VW. VWD **can be acquired** and a history of medications, notably anticonvulsants, is important. Most spontaneous emergencies (i.e., other than those due to trauma) will be in patients with severe disease. For patients with known VWD who present with bleeding, management depends on the severity and type of bleeding as well as the type of VWD but includes:

- Local methods with pressure for epistaxis and fibrin sealants, or the use of anti-fibrinolytics (amicar [50 mg/kg q6hr IV or PO with a max dose of 5 g q6hr] or tranexamic acid [Lysteda 20–40 mg/kg/d div bid or tid max dose of 1,300 mg q8hr PO]). **Contraindications to anti-fibrinolytic use** include the presence of hematuria, DIC, or increased thrombotic risk;

- For heavy menstrual bleeding, hormonal control can be used. This usually will be with estrogen-containing medications unless there are contraindications such as a personal or family history of clots, breast cancer, and arguably in patients with vascular malformations. You may want help from Gynecology if such bleeding is a major overnight issue;

- For type 1 VWD patients, if these measures are insufficient DDAVP (desmopressin) can be given subcutaneously or IV (0.3 mcg/kg) no more than once daily. More frequent administration can lead to fluid overload, hyponatremia, and potentially seizures, particularly in very young children (<3 years of age). Stimate (intranasal DDAVP) is not currently available in many centers;

- DDAVP may not be effective in a subset of type 1 patients and is not effective in any patients with types 2 or 3. In these patients, for uncontrolled bleeding episodes VWF:Ristocetin cofactor concentrate or recombinant VWF (Humate [VWF, F8 complex] is a good place to start with an initial dose of 40–60 IU/kg based on

DOI: 10.1201/9781003473701-33

VWF not factor 8 content) for major bleeding episodes. If these are not available, you can use cryoprecipitate (which contains both VWF and factor 8 protein);

- If a patient is being sent home from the ER, be sure the family has access to replacement factors or antifibrinolytics which often are not easily available at local pharmacies. Follow-up with a *hemophilia* treatment center or bleeding clinic needs to be arranged for teaching (including genetic counseling) and management.

Bibliography

Callaghan MU, Wong TE, Federici AB. Treatment of acquired von Willebrand syndrome in childhood. *Blood*. 2013;122:2019–2022.

What ChatGPT Says

Not much granularity to this relating to acute management but worth mentioning that at least in the US, **Stimate (nasal DDAVP) has not been available for some time**.

1. *Management*:
   a. *Desmopressin (DDAVP) therapy*:
      - DDAVP is a medication that can be used to treat mild to moderate forms of VWD, particularly type 1 and some cases of type 2. It works by releasing stored VWF from endothelial cells and increasing VWF and factor VIII levels in the blood.
      - DDAVP can be administered intravenously or intranasally, and its effectiveness should be tested to ensure an appropriate response.
   b. *Replacement therapy*:
      - Children with more severe VWD or those who do not respond to DDAVP may require replacement therapy with VWF-containing concentrates. These concentrates may contain both VWF and factor VIII and can be used to prevent or treat bleeding episodes.
      - The dosing and frequency of replacement therapy depend on the child's specific VWD type, severity, and clinical situation.
   c. *Menstrual management*:
      - Adolescent girls with VWD may experience heavy or prolonged menstrual bleeding. This can be managed with medications, such as hormonal therapy or tranexamic acid, to reduce bleeding during menstruation.

Algorithm: VWD and Other Factor Deficiencies

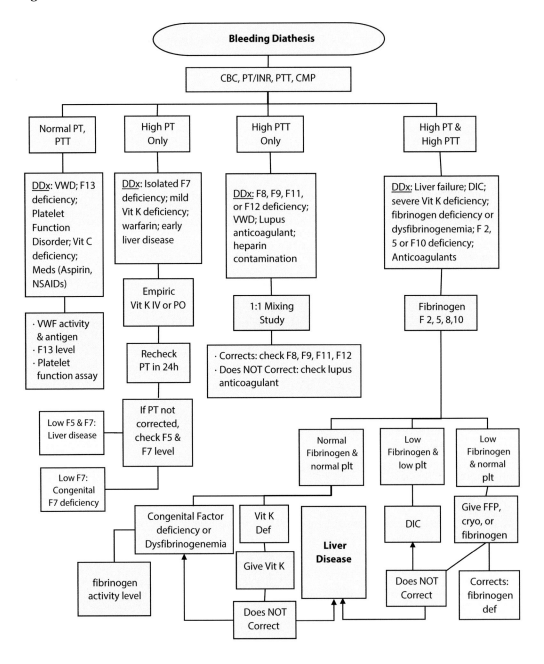

32

Vitamin K Deficiency

Vitamin K deficiency can present with bleeding at any age, usually of skin and mucous membranes but can cause serious internal bleeding. The most common causes of vitamin K deficiency are dietary (poor intake) and antibiotic interference with normal gut flora and absorption. Less common causes are cystic fibrosis with deficiencies of the vitamins ADEK. Newborns have low vitamin K and should get vitamin K shots in the delivery room to avoid hemorrhagic disease of the newborn (*Neonatal Hematologic Emergencies*). Laboratory evaluation (*Bleeding Emergencies*) will show elevated PT/INR but not always an elevated PTT (both correct with 1:1 mix), and low plasma levels of factors 2, 7, 9, 10—**factor 7 has the shortest half-life so is the most sensitive**. **PIVKA** (proteins induced by vitamin K absence) is a functional marker of vitamin K status, but worry about this electively. Genetically driven isolated factor 7 deficiency or dysfunction can be seen without vitamin K deficiency. Overnight, **if vitamin K deficiency is suspected, consider treating even if only the INR and PTT are resulted and factor levels are still pending**. Intravenous vitamin K (see the Harriet Lane *Handbook* or Micromedex for dosing) should improve coagulation studies within 24 hours, but ongoing treatment may be needed. Deal with that in the morning.

What ChatGPT Says

A pretty generic response and not much help for the rare night-time emergency but appropriate mention of dietary sources of vitamin K—leafy green vegetables (such as spinach, kale, and broccoli), brussels sprouts, cabbage, asparagus, and fermented foods like natto—is made.

1. *Diagnosis*:
   a. *Clinical assessment*: … conduct a thorough clinical assessment, including obtaining a detailed dietary history and performing a physical examination. Symptoms may include easy bruising, mucosal bleeding (e.g., nosebleeds, bleeding gums), and, in severe cases, spontaneous internal bleeding.

DOI: 10.1201/9781003473701-34

b. *Laboratory tests*:
- *Prothrombin time (PT) and international normalized ratio (INR)*: These tests evaluate blood clotting function and may show prolonged clotting times in cases of vitamin K deficiency.
- *Vitamin K levels*: Measuring vitamin K levels in the blood can help confirm the deficiency.
- *Liver function tests*: Vitamin K is absorbed in the intestines and requires normal liver function for activation. Liver function tests may be performed to assess liver health.

c. *Underlying causes*: Determine the underlying cause of vitamin K deficiency, which could be due to inadequate dietary intake, malabsorption issues, or underlying medical conditions.

2. *Management*:

The management of vitamin K deficiency in childhood involves several components, depending on the severity and underlying cause:

a. *Dietary changes*:
- In cases of dietary vitamin K deficiency, improving the child's diet by including foods rich in vitamin K, such as green leafy vegetables (e.g., spinach, kale, broccoli), can help correct the deficiency.

b. *Vitamin K supplementation*:
- For moderate to severe cases of vitamin K deficiency or in cases of malabsorption, vitamin K supplementation is often necessary. This can be administered orally or intravenously, depending on the severity of the deficiency.

c. *Treatment of underlying causes*:
- If the deficiency is caused by malabsorption issues, gastrointestinal disorders, or liver disease, the underlying condition should be treated and managed accordingly.

Algorithm: **see chapter 31**

33

Other Factor Deficiencies

Other factor deficiencies present pretty much like *hemophilia* or *VWD* and should be suspected based on family history or when either the PT, PTT, or occasionally both are abnormal and correct with 1:1 mixing studies. Levels in deficient patients may not correspond to bleeding risk: Some patients with very low levels may not bleed whereas others with milder deficiencies (higher levels) may bleed. Factor 12 deficiency causes prolonged PTT but does not usually cause bleeding. **Factor 13 deficiency is a rare bird that should be thought of when PT, PTT, and platelet levels are normal** in patients with delayed bleeding, poor wound healing, or intracranial hemorrhage. Confirmation of specific factor deficiencies requires measurement of levels in venous or umbilical vein blood. These usually result quickly (within a few hours) in a tertiary care center (except for Factor 13 which is usually a send-out lab). **Routine coagulation studies generally are normal until individual factor levels are <30%.** The good news is that spontaneous bleeding doesn't usually occur with mild factor deficiencies. Treatment requires an understanding of what products contain what factors (recombinant factors are not universally available):

Product	Contents
Cryoprecipitate	F8,13, Fibrinogen, VWF, ADAMTS13
FFP	all pro- and anti-coagulants
Recombinant Fibrinogen (Fibryga)	Fibrinogen
Humate	VWF, F8

Bibliography

Jain S, Acharya SS. Management of rare coagulation disorders in 2018. *Transfus Apher Sci.* 2018;57: 705–712.

Peyvandi F, Jayandharan G, Chandy M, et al. Genetic diagnosis of haemophilia and other inherited bleeding disorders. *Haemophilia* 2006;12(Suppl 3):82–89.

DOI: 10.1201/9781003473701-35

What ChatGPT Says

We queried each of the miscellaneous factor deficiencies and ChatGPT didn't say much; it's not worth taking up space with what it did include.

Algorithm: **see chapter 31**

34

Neonatal Hematologic Emergencies

Several of the night-time emergencies that are seen in neonates are discussed in earlier sections (*Massive Hepatomegaly, Hemolytic Anemia, Arterial Strokes, Vitamin K Deficiency*, and *Other Factor Deficiencies*). When evaluating bleeding or thrombosis in neonates (<1 month of age for term babies) or infants (≤1 year of age), the first order of business is to recognize that "normative" values are very different from what they are in older children. Have 24-7 access to texts such as the Harriet Lane *Handbook* or the appendices of *Nathan and Oski*! In general, coagulation factors and pro-thrombotic factors such as Protein C and S are low except for factors 5, 8, 13, VWF, and fibrinogen (which after 32 weeks' gestation are the same as in adults), leading to normally "increased" aPTT and PT/INR levels compared to older children and adults. These factors do not cross the placenta but most will reach adult levels by 6 months of age. Increased levels of VWF, along with decreased production of both pro- and anti-thrombotic proteins create a balanced hemostatic system in neonates. Look to be sure you know if baby is a boy or a girl, since some coag abnormalities are X-linked. Platelet numbers are about what they are in older children and adults, although levels as low as 80,000/mm³ occasionally can be seen in otherwise normal neonates. Platelet function is generally less good than at older ages and there are no good normative values for platelet function assays (PFA)—elevated levels may not be diagnostic of platelet dysfunction in children under a year of age. Haptoglobin levels also are normally "low" in neonates. Very *high WBC* in newborns, especially in those with Down syndrome may signal **transient myeloproliferative syndrome**. So—management works backward from labs:

- CBC diff, MCV, PT, PTT; hypercoagulation workup as indicated;
  - Looking at newborn peripheral blood smears is an art form that you probably won't master on-call, but you should at least be able to confirm platelet size and the absence of clumping. If there is a question of **pseudo-thrombocytopenia**, recheck a blood draw in sodium citrate or heparin. Schistocytes are not always pathologic, especially in babies;
  - Most syndromes involving platelets can be discussed on morning rounds but if bleeding occurs in the face of normal numbers of large platelets, have platelets ready for *transfusion emergencies*. **Most centers require type & cross for newborns and maybe even two samples** before transfusion of any blood products;
  - If a factor deficiency is suspected (e.g., in male neonates where the mother is a known hemophilia carrier), send a stat cord blood sample for factor level;
  - Remember that **early exposure to factor products, as in newborns, encourages the development of inhibitors. Avoid where possible**;
  - If a left-shifted *high WBC* w/wo low platelets suggests myeloproliferation, consider getting a peripheral blood karyotype to look for Trisomy 21;
  - Rare but an emergency is congenital TTP or **Upshaw–Shulman syndrome**;

DOI: 10.1201/9781003473701-36

- Physical examination, to document VS and whether the baby looks ill, plus type and extent of bleeding with a complete skin exam. Look for organomegaly, fontanelle status, cephalohematoma, and neurologic status, especially focality to suggest a stroke; dysmorphisms that might suggest Down syndrome or other trisomies, thrombocytopenia absent radii (TAR) syndrome, or even weirder syndromes; obvious *vascular malformations* or vascular tumors including congenital hemangiomas and Kaposiform hemangioendothelioma;
- History of familial platelet or coag problems: maternal ITP (document mom's platelet count at delivery and in her past) or HELLP, intrauterine medication exposure, neonatal issues in older sibs; intrauterine infections (TORCHS, HIV, sepsis), fetal distress; had baby undergone ECMO;
  - Did baby get vitamin K in the delivery room? If not, beware of **hemorrhagic disease of the newborn** due to *Vitamin K deficiency*, especially as some families are declining this intervention;
- No night-time circumcisions if any question of coagulopathy**, in which case, also avoid IM shots (Vitamin K can be given subq**; Hep B should be delayed until there is a definitive coag deficiency diagnosis) or if there is active concern for Hep B—in those cases, give IM and **hold pressure** for 5 minutes. Same for heel stick sites;
- Whether imaging is needed urgently is usually a neonatal intensive care unit (NICU) or PICU decision but newborn **ultrasounds of the head** to look for bleeds are considered to be accurate until age 6 months. Anything in the head—call a Neurology consult.

Bibliography

Anderson CC, Kapoor S, Mark TE, eds, *The Harriet Lane Handbook*, 23rd edn, Elsevier 2023.

Dunbar M, Kirton A. Perinatal stroke: Mechanisms, management, and outcomes of early cerebrovascular brain injury. *Lancet Child Adolesc Health*. 2018;2:666–676.

Ferriero DM, Fullerton HJ, Bernard TJ, et al. Management of stroke in neonates and children: A scientific statement from the American Heart Association/American Stroke Association. *Stroke*. 2019;50:e51–e96.

Orkin SH, Nathan DG, Ginsburg D, et al., eds, *Nathan and Oski's Hematology and Oncology of Infancy and Childhood*, 8nd edn, Elsevier 2014.

What ChatGPT Says

We didn't check more detailed queries and these may give better answers, but what we found was too generic to be worth taking space to report.

Algorithm: **see** *Massive Hepatomegaly, Hemolytic Anemia, Arterial Strokes, Vitamin K Deficiency,* **and** *Other Factor Deficiencies*

35

COVID-19 and Hematologic Emergencies

Although COVID-19 had appeared to be on the wane, clearly we are still seeing it, especially in unvaccinated and other at-risk immunocompromised individuals such as those typically seen on PHO in-patient services. Children most commonly will be admitted to a general pediatric floor or PICU but you may be consulted overnight, usually with questions relating to **COVID as a hypercoaguable state**. COVID-19 is well-known to increase the risk for VTE in children as well as adults, and thromboembolic events have occurred with COVID-19 despite prophylactic anticoagulation (ppx). Children ≥12 years old have a significantly higher risk for thrombosis compared to that of the normal population with both COVID-19 or the closely related multisystem inflammatory syndrome in children (MIS-C). Elevated D-dimer levels tend to portend a worse prognosis. The NIH recommends that any child ≥12 years old who is admitted for COVID-19 receive ppx, although others have used a more individualized approach based on **risk factors in addition to age and post-pubertal status and COVID severity**: central venous catheter; on a ventilator; an anticipated hospital stay of more than 3 days; immobility; obesity; known thrombophilia with or without prior history of *DVT* or *PE*; active malignancy or nephrotic syndrome; cystic fibrosis or *SCD crisis*; flare of underlying inflammatory conditions; congenital heart disease with venous stasis; first-degree family history of VTE; estrogen-containing birth control. Whether anti-platelet therapy such as daily baby aspirin is needed is, in our center, determined by cardiology and/or rheumatology. Follow up with CBC diff and DIC panel the next day and decide on other monitoring including discharge planning on morning rounds. Someone needs to determine whether to treat the underlying COVID, but probably not PHO. Remember: On occasion, **COVID vaccination has been associated with thrombocytopenia or thrombosis**. Whether anti-platelet therapy such as daily baby aspirin is needed is, in our center, determined by cardiology and/or rheumatology. Follow-up CBC diff, DIC panel the next day, and rest of monitoring, decide on rounds. What happens after discharge can be planned on days. Someone needs to remember to **treat** COVID-19, but probably not PHO. A diagnosis of COVID-19 in any pediatric in-patient is enough to trigger an evaluation and decision-making regarding the need for ppx or treatment doses of anticoagulation.

Bibliography

Iba T, Levy JH. Thrombosis and thrombocytopenia in COVID-19 and after COVID-19 vaccination. *Trends Cardiovasc Med.* 2022;32:249–256.

DOI: 10.1201/9781003473701-37

Loi M, Branchford B, Kim J, et al. Covid-19 anticoagulation recommendations in children. *Pediatr Blood Cancer*. 2020;67(9):e28485.

NIH, Therapeutic Management of Hospitalized Children with Covid-19, 2022. Available at: https://www.covid19treatmentguidelines.nih.gov/management/clinical-management-of-children/hospitalized-children-therapeutic-management

Whitworth H, Sartain SE, Kumar R, et al. Rate of thrombosis in children and adolescents hospitalized with Covid-19 or MIS-C. *Blood* 2021;138(2):190–198.

What ChatGPT Says

Not bad as an overview, but vague.

Hematologic emergencies in the context of a COVID-19 infection can occur as a result of the virus's impact on various components of the blood and the coagulation system. These emergencies can have serious consequences and may include conditions such as thrombosis, bleeding disorders, and changes in blood cell counts. Here are some hematologic emergencies associated with COVID-19:

1. *Thrombosis and hypercoagulability*: COVID-19 has been linked to an increased risk of blood clot formation, including deep vein thrombosis (DVT), pulmonary embolism (PE), stroke, and other thrombotic events. These events can be life-threatening and require prompt treatment with anticoagulants.

2. *Disseminated intravascular coagulation (DIC)*: Some severe cases of COVID-19 can trigger a condition called DIC, where the body's normal clotting mechanisms become overactive, leading to widespread clot formation. This can lead to bleeding complications and organ damage.

3. *Thrombocytopenia*: A drop in platelet counts (thrombocytopenia) can occur in COVID-19 patients, leading to an increased risk of bleeding. It's important to monitor platelet counts and manage thrombocytopenia accordingly.

4. *Immune thrombocytopenic purpura (ITP)*: There have been reports of ITP occurring after COVID-19 vaccination or infection, where the immune system mistakenly attacks and destroys platelets. Treatment may involve immunosuppressive medications.

5. *Hemorrhagic complications*: Severe COVID-19 cases can sometimes lead to bleeding complications, such as gastrointestinal bleeding, intracranial hemorrhage, or other forms of spontaneous bleeding. These may require treatment and supportive care.

6. *Anemia*: COVID-19 can cause anemia due to various mechanisms, including inflammation, bone marrow suppression, and hemolysis. Managing anemia may involve addressing the underlying cause and providing transfusions if necessary.

7. *Neutropenia and leukopenia*: COVID-19 can affect white blood cell counts, including neutrophils (neutropenia) and overall white blood cell counts (leukopenia). Monitoring for infections and providing appropriate treatment is essential.

8. *Hematologic malignancies*: COVID-19 can be particularly challenging for individuals with hematologic malignancies such as leukemia or lymphoma, as it can weaken the immune system and complicate treatment.

Algorithm: COVID and Hematologic Emergencies

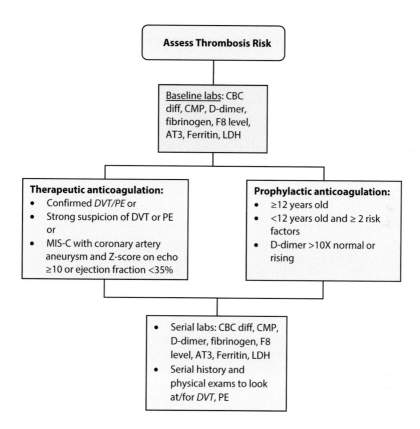

36

Hemophagocytic Lympho-Histiocytosis (HLH)

Hemophagocytic lympho-histiocytosis (HLH) is a symptom complex that looks like a lot of other diseases (or they look like HLH). Some patients are very ill and for that reason you will get called even on nights to help with evaluations and weigh in on treatment. The diagnosis involves suspicion based on context (family history of HLH or similar symptoms, malignancy, infection or post-vaccination, rheumatoid disease), a menu of clinical and laboratory variables including fever (>38.5°), more than one cytopenia, splenomegaly, hyperferritinemia (>500 ng/mL), hypertriglyceridemia, hypofibrinogenemia, hemophagocytosis on tissue biopsy, elevated soluble IL2 receptor (sIL2R) levels. Although five of these technically are required for diagnosis (hepatomegaly, while common, is not a criterion), findings often evolve and can be atypical. Primary HLH refers to a genetic or strongly suspected genetic component (e.g., perforin, SAP, XIAP, or CD107a deficiency). Secondary HLH is everything else. Night-time emergencies require symptom control, suspicion of the diagnosis, thinking about differential diagnosis (malignancy, infection, macrophage activating syndrome [MAS] which is now often labeled HLH-MAS in patients with underlying rheumatoid disease), starting the evaluation, and occasionally starting decadron (10 mg/m^2 IV or PO daily with consideration of duration and addition of other agents to follow in the AM). The only cure for primary HLH is a stem cell transplant—not one for on-call initiation! Blood for genetic testing or "send-out" HLH panels that include relevant genes can be drawn but usually not until the next morning, Monday–Friday.

Bibliography

Canna SW, Marsh RA. Pediatric hemophagocytic lymphohistiocytosis. *Blood*. 2020;135:1332–1343.

Emile JF, Abla O, Fraitag S, et al. Revised classification of histiocytoses and neoplasms of the macrophage-dendritic cell lineages. *Blood*. 2016;127:2672–2681.

Henter JI, Horne A, Aricó M, et al. HOH-2004: Diagnostic and therapeutic guidelines for hemophagocytic lymphohistiocytosis. *Pediatr Blood Cancer*. 2007;48:124–131.

DOI: 10.1201/9781003473701-38

What ChatGPT Says

Not a bad overview but not detailed enough for overnight efficiency:

Hemophagocytic lymphohistiocytosis (HLH) is a rare and potentially life-threatening immune disorder that affects the body's ability to control the immune response. It is characterized by an uncontrolled activation of certain immune cells called T cells and macrophages, leading to excessive inflammation and tissue damage. HLH can be classified into two main forms:

1. *Primary HLH*: This form is inherited and typically appears in early childhood. It is caused by genetic mutations affecting proteins involved in immune regulation, such as perforin, MUNC13-4, STX11, STXBP2, and others.

2. *Secondary HLH*: This form can occur at any age and is usually triggered by infections (e.g., viral infectious ones like Epstein–Barr virus), autoimmune disorders, or malignancies (e.g., lymphomas). The symptoms of HLH can include fever, enlarged liver and spleen, cytopenias (low blood cell counts, including anemia, low platelets, and low white blood cells), and other signs of organ dysfunction. Diagnosing HLH can be challenging due to its nonspecific symptoms and rarity. It often requires a combination of clinical evaluation, blood tests, bone marrow examination, and genetic testing to determine the specific form of HLH. The treatment for HLH usually involves suppressing the overactive immune system using medications like corticosteroids, immunosuppressive drugs (e.g., etoposide), and sometimes other targeted therapies like interleukin-1 (IL-1) or interleukin-6 (IL-6) inhibitors. In severe cases, hematopoietic stem cell transplantation may be considered for primary HLH.

Algorithm: **Hemophagocytic Lympho-Histiocytosis (HLH)**[*]

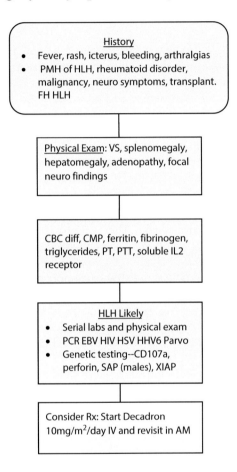

History
- Fever, rash, icterus, bleeding, arthralgias
- PMH of HLH, rheumatoid disorder, malignancy, neuro symptoms, transplant. FH HLH

Physical Exam: VS, splenomegaly, hepatomegaly, adenopathy, focal neuro findings

CBC diff, CMP, ferritin, fibrinogen, triglycerides, PT, PTT, soluble IL2 receptor

HLH Likely
- Serial labs and physical exam
- PCR EBV HIV HSV HHV6 Parvo
- Genetic testing--CD107a, perforin, SAP (males), XIAP

Consider Rx: Start Decadron 10mg/m^2/day IV and revisit in AM

---

[*] see Canna and Henter references for additional algorithms

Part III

Vascular Anomalies

Vascular anomalies (VA) include vascular tumors such as hemangiomas and vascular malformations that can involve any combination of veins, arteries, lymphatics, and capillaries. These mostly are elective daytime issues (think about that when you are looking for a career subspecialty within PHO) but we include here a few references and scenarios relating to emergencies you may encounter when you are on-call. A classification scheme for thinking about VA can be found at www.issva.org.

Bibliography

DeMaio A, New C, Bergmann S. Medical Treatment of Vascular Anomalies. *Dermatol Clin.* 2022;40:461–471.

International Society for the Study of Vascular Anomalies: https://ISSVA.org

Mack JM, Crary SE. How we approach coagulopathy with vascular anomalies. *Pediatr Blood Cancer.* 2022;69(Suppl 3):e29353. doi:10.1002/pbc.29353.

Nakano TA, Dori Y, Gumer L, et al. How we approach pediatric congenital chylous effusions and ascites. *Pediatr Blood Cancer.* 2022;Suppl 3:e29246.

Serio J, Gattoline S, Collier H, Bustin A. Evaluation of Sirolimus dosing in neonates and infants with lymphatic disorders: A case series. 2022;27:447–451.

DOI: 10.1201/9781003473701-39

37

Pain in Vascular Anomalies

In most cases, the on-call fellow will hear about this when a parent calls from home, and will need to decide whether the patient needs to come to the ER urgently. In other cases, it may be the ER calling to say that the patient needs to be admitted for pain management. In many cases, this will be a fellow's first experience with VA and, as these are not so rare as you may think, this is a good opportunity to learn about these disorders. Pain is more common in patients with VM (vascular malformations) than in those with vascular tumors and may be due to acute exacerbation of swelling of the lesion (due to systemic or local infection, trauma, or "just because") or more likely due to local intralesional coagulation (LIC) since a VM is a hypercoagulable state. Although LIC occasionally can lead to pulmonary emboli (PE) or strokes, LIC is generally not lethal. However, the degree of pain may be enough to keep a fellow awake at night. A few suggestions may help with management, and ideally with keeping the patient at home until the clinic is open:

- If the child is followed by a vascular anomalies specialist, review a recent note that may well include guidelines about management;
- Take a quick history: Is the child so sick that he/she/they sound septic, or is chest pain so severe and associated with shortness of breath to suggest a PE and need for immediate attention? If not, be sure that the pain is in an area related to a known VM; ask family whether this has happened before, what was done then and now, and what has worked; has the patient had a recent procedure such as sclerotherapy which can cause LIC or thrombophlebitis; ask about redness overlying the VM that might suggest *cellulitis*; what medicines is the patient taking?
- Physical examination on-site or by a parent at home: is there more than the usual swelling, overlying redness or blue lymphatic blebs, tenderness to palpation? Are there hard areas within the area of VM—these may be phleboliths ("stones") that indicate LIC? Try to ensure that there is no other reason for the pain—these patients can break legs and arms, get appendicitis, etc., as well as anyone else;
- If not already done—try ice packs (for most patients ice is better than heat) and ibuprofen (age-based dose on high end, q6 hour for no more than 2 days to minimize ibuprofen-related renal issues)—most likely all of these interventions will have been done before the family called but maybe not;
- If the patient is at the hospital, consider drawing blood for d-dimers, fibrinogen, CBC with platelet count, and maybe PT (INR) and PTT that may establish a new baseline. Normal levels do not exclude LIC and abnormal levels are not diagnostic—but they support the diagnosis. Compare with prior labs if any;

DOI: 10.1201/9781003473701-40

- There is **no need for middle-of-the-night PVLs** or other radiographs for localized pain related to VM;
- Several options that can be elected outpatient or inpatient:
  - One is to start steroids—and one option is prednisone 1 mg/kg PO bid (we often max at 40–60 mg a day depending on patient size) for 2 days with a taper over a week—remember, all you need to do is get the patient through until the next morning. The only catch is to be sure that if the family is home, there is a local pharmacy that is open at night. Improvement may take a few days;
  - Another is to start prophylactic anticoagulation. Lovenox (LMWH) is not usually an option for first-time users as an outpatient in the middle of the night but DOACs notably Xarelto are increasingly being used for this purpose in prophylactic doses without loading. 10–20 mg a day is usually adequate with responses within a week or two. These medicines won't work if the pharmacy can't fill the prescription at night (or if copay is too high);
    - Be sure there is no other bleeding diathesis, and menarchal females may need to hold dose during periods—so timing is key;
  - More therapy targeted to the VM such as sirolimus may help prevent these issues in the future but this is not a middle-of-the-night thing for outpatients;
  - Standard pain meds such as gabapentin and even narcotics frequently are not effective;
- If the patient remains an outpatient, be sure the family calls its vascular anomalies doc the next working day;
- Consider antibiotics if there is concern for *cellulitis*: ampicillin or clindamycin.

What ChatGPT Says

As expected for this area that is a relatively new addition to PHO, nothing much is available on ChatGPT. We were impressed that in contrast to searches we did several months ago, there actually were some attempts to address diagnosis and management issues. This is likely to improve over time and you may want to revisit.

Algorithm: Pain in Vascular Anomalies

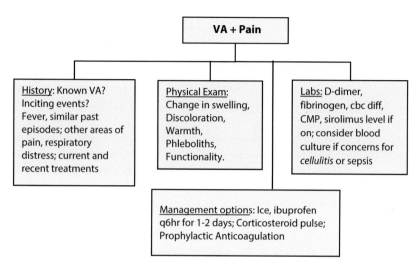

38

Cellulitis vs. Inflammation in Vascular Anomalies

Redness of the skin over a VM is usually seen in patients with lymphatic malformations and cutaneous "blebs" who often have an overlying capillary malformation. Inflammation is probably more common than infection (cellulitis) but this can be a difficult distinction, especially in very young babies. If in doubt, a blood culture with IV or IM ceftriaxone and/ or oral antibiotics (clindamycin, or augmentin if available) is reasonable. Lab work (see *Pain*) in addition to blood culture is worthwhile as a baseline but won't distinguish these possibilities. These interventions are usually done from the ER as outpatients but you may get called, and if a child looks sick, we suggest admission for observation and ongoing antibiotics. Oral corticosteroids (prednisone or decadron pulse, as described for pain) can ameliorate pain. Before sending a patient home, be sure that there is a pharmacy where prescriptions can be filled and that there is follow-up with PCP or vascular anomalies clinic.

What ChatGPT Says

As expected for this area that is a relatively new addition to PHO, nothing much is available on ChatGPT. We were impressed that in contrast to searches we did several months ago, there actually were some attempts to address diagnosis and management issues. This is likely to improve over time and you may want to revisit.

DOI: 10.1201/9781003473701-41

39

Effusions with/without Organ Failure in Vascular Anomalies

Effusions in most pediatric settings are exudative effusions or edema due to congestive heart failure, nephrotic syndrome or liver failure having nothing to do with vascular anomalies. PHO usually will not be the primary team overnight. However, there is a good chance you will get called in consultation once lymphatic (chylous) effusions are identified. Chylous ascites, pleural or pericardial effusions can be initial or ongoing presentations of syndromes such as Noonan syndrome or other causes of central conducting lymphatic anomaly (CCLA). Isolated lymphedema without effusions is more likely in Down syndrome or Turner syndrome. Although not problems that can be solved overnight, keeping these entities on your radar and some initial interventions can minimize complications. Much of the workup probably will have been done before you are called:

- Imaging to define location and extent of effusions: CXR, ultrasound, echocardiogram as clinically indicated; MRI with and without contrast can help distinguish between chyle and non-chylous effusions;

- History to look at the progression of signs and symptoms including swelling, distention, and respiratory distress; known history of vascular anomalies or syndromes known to be associated with effusions; history of infections that can exacerbate effusions;

- Physical examination: VS including O_2 saturation;

- Laboratory studies should include CBC diff (mostly to look for platelet counts and lymphopenia), CMP including albumin and total protein, and IgG levels—all of these can be low in such patients; d-dimers, fibrinogen, and stool alpha-1 antitrypsin if protein-losing enteropathy suspected;

- Although asymptomatic patients can be watched, they are not the patients who are admitted. For patients with symptomatic effusions:
  - Consult VIR or surgery to place a drain—fluid analysis will show high triglycerides in patients with chylous effusions (>110 mg/dL). Often these are milky white. This is likely a job best done in the PICU;
  - Measure the rate of fluid leak to determine the severity of disease, which may direct management (>20 mL/kg/day is a high rate and will usually need more treatment in light of day);

DOI: 10.1201/9781003473701-42

- Overnight, it may be easiest to make the patient NPO and put on a medium-chain triglyceride (MCT) diet, replete albumin and electrolytes with lasix diuresis (just a temporizing plan for patients with high rates of re-accumulation since these problems will recur without definitive treatment);
- Rarely, octreotide infusions are initiated on nights, but that is the PICU's job, not yours.

What ChatGPT Says

Although AI doesn't address vascular anomalies as an etiology, it is not bad about a more generic approach to chylous effusions:

1. *Identify and treat the underlying cause*: Chylous effusions are usually secondary to an underlying condition such as trauma, malignancy, or certain medical procedures. Identifying and treating the primary cause is essential for effective management. This may involve surgery, radiation therapy, or medications, depending on the specific condition.

2. *Symptom management*: Chylous effusions can cause symptoms like shortness of breath, cough, and chest pain. Symptomatic relief can be achieved through various methods, including:

   a. *Thoracentesis or paracentesis*: Draining the accumulated fluid can help relieve symptoms and improve respiratory function.

   b. *Dietary modifications*: A low-fat diet with medium-chain triglycerides (MCT) can reduce the production of chyle. Avoiding long-chain triglycerides (LCT) found in foods like dairy products, eggs, and fatty meats can help. Consult a registered dietitian for appropriate dietary recommendations.

   c. *Nutritional support*: In severe cases, total parenteral nutrition (TPN) or enteral nutrition may be required to provide adequate nutrition while minimizing the intake of fat.

   d. *Medications*: Medications such as somatostatin analogs (e.g., octreotide) or fibrin sealants (e.g., talc slurry) may be used in some cases to reduce chyle production or promote the closure of leaky lymphatic vessels.

Algorithm: Effusions with/without Organ Failure

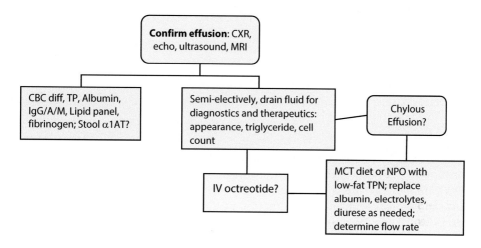

40

Pulmonary Embolus in Patients with Vascular Malformations

Initial management of Pulmonary embolus is the same as that for PE in other settings. This complication is not seen that we know of in the setting of vascular tumors. Follow-up attention to the LIC, which is the underlying cause of PE in patients with vascular malformations, can be dealt with in the setting of a multidisciplinary vascular anomalies clinic. Patients with VM and PE also may have *pain*.

What ChatGPT Says

See *Pulmonary Embolus*, Chapter 24.

Algorithm chapter 24

DOI: 10.1201/9781003473701-43

41

Kasabach–Merritt Phenomenon in Vascular Anomalies

Kasabach–Merritt Phenomenon (KMP) is the association of low platelets (<50,000/mm^3), low fibrinogen (often <100 mg/dL), prolonged INR and PTT, elevated D-dimers often with mucocutaneous or deep bleeding. In the context of VA, KMP is seen in patients with kaposiform hemangioendothelioma (KHE, synonymous with tufted angioma), or with kaposiform lymphatic anomaly (KLA). These are diagnoses that can be difficult to make even with experience, but think about them when there are the lab abnormalities noted above. KHE can occur at any age but presents most commonly in early infancy especially as a superficial indurated purple-colored mass, more commonly in girls and on the trunk or extremities—but can occur internally. **Don't** be tempted to biopsy these lesions unless you have backup from Interventional Radiology as they can bleed profusely. **Don't** be tempted to replace clotting factors repeatedly since that may make the consumption worse—although major bleeding may require factor replacement. If you do transfuse platelets, check 1-hour counts (*Thrombocytopenia with/without Bleeding*). Definitive treatment usually starts with high-dose prednisone (≥1 mg/kg IV methylprednisolone bid) but sirolimus alone or in addition to steroids may be the easiest next step. Because sirolimus dosing is both age and size-based, it may be easier for clinicians with less experience to start on days. One recent reference suggested a starting dose of 0.5 mg/m^2/day given as a once-daily dose for patients <1 year of age, and many use 8 mg/m^2 PO bid for patients 1–18 years. Older patients often are started on a dose of 2 mg a day. IV vincristine (0.05 mg/kg max 2.4 mg) is probably as good as sirolimus but ideally requires a central line in babies and children.

What ChatGPT Says

ChatGPT is okay on this topic, although we would not support propranolol as an intervention.

The treatment of Kasabach–Merritt phenomenon in the context of KHE can be challenging and may require a multidisciplinary approach involving pediatricians, hematologists, and surgeons. Treatment options may include:

1. *Medical management*:
   a. *Corticosteroids*: High doses of corticosteroids can be used to help shrink the tumor and improve platelet counts.
   b. *Vincristine*: This medication can be used to disrupt the tumor's blood vessels and decrease platelet trapping.

DOI: 10.1201/9781003473701-44

2. *Interventional radiology*:
   a. *Embolization*: Embolization procedures involve blocking the blood vessels supplying the tumor, which can reduce bleeding and size.
3. *Surgery*:
   a. In some cases, surgical removal of the tumor might be considered, especially if the tumor is causing severe complications.
4. *Other therapies*:
   a. *Sirolimus*: This medication has been used to manage vascular anomalies and might be considered in certain cases.
   b. *Propranolol*: In some instances, propranolol, a beta-blocker, has been used to help manage KHE.
5. *Supportive care*:
   a. Blood and platelet transfusions might be necessary to manage bleeding and thrombocytopenia.

Algorithm: **Kasabach–Merritt Phenomenon**

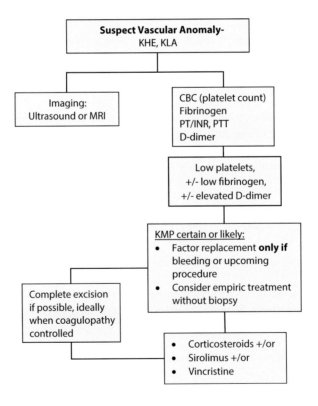

Part IV

General

42

Managing Symptoms at the End of Life

The active stage of dying can last days to weeks. It is characterized by decreased responsiveness, changes in vital signs (bradycardia, hypotension, hypoxia), respiratory changes (irregular, shallow, episodes of apnea, inability to manage airway secretions), decreased perfusion (coolness and mottling of extremities), and changes in urinary and stool output. Anticipatory counseling for the family is indicated, and ideally should be provided electively by team members best known to the family. The key to management of acute or progressive symptoms is anticipation (see *What To Do When a Patient Dies*, Chapter 43).

- Be sure you know the patient's DNR status **before** you assume care. Even if a patient clearly is dying, no code status documentation obligates the staff to call a code in the event of clinical deterioration;
- Know who wants or needs to be notified in the event of clinical deterioration and death;
- It is not a bad idea to know whether autopsy and funeral arrangements have been discussed;
- Problems that may require attention overnight include:
  - Air hunger:
    - Opioids (first line)
      - Opioid dosing for air hunger is generally 25–50% less than that required for pain (see next)
    - Benzodiazepines can be used as adjunctive agents for anxiety associated with dyspnea
      - Lorazepam 0.1 mg/kg PO, sublingual (SL), or IV
    - A fan to the face may relieve dyspnea but its use is restricted in many hospital settings;
    - Avoid supplemental oxygen unless it provides symptomatic relief;
    - A blender with 21% FiO_2 can be used to deliver flow without providing additional oxygen;
  - Anxiety:
    - Benzodiazepines (first line);
      - Lorazepam 0.1 mg/kg PO, SL, or IV;
    - Treat underlying pain and other symptoms;

DOI: 10.1201/9781003473701-46

- Delirium (confusion and changes in level of consciousness):
  - Non-pharmacologic interventions (redirection, talking to the patient, maintaining a distinction between days and night);
  - Melatonin at night can be helpful if sleep disruption is a contributing factor;
  - Pharmacologic management (atypical antipsychotics):
    - Risperidone 0.1–0.2 mg nightly (children <5 years); 0.2–0.5 mg nightly (children ≥5 years)
    - Olanzapine 1.25–5 mg daily or twice daily (children ≥3 years)
    - Quetiapine 0.5 mg/kg/dose q8–12 hours
- Pain:
  - Dosing of opioids at the end of life is impacted by a patient's opioid requirement in the weeks prior. Patients receiving chronic opioids should, at minimum, be started on doses equivalent to their baseline usage;
  - The following are typical starting doses for opioid-naïve patients:
    - Oral route
      - Morphine 0.2–0.5 mg/kg/dose q3–4 h PO or SL
      - Hydromorphone 0.03–0.08 mg/kg/dose q3–4 h PO
      - Oxycodone 0.1–0.2 mg/kg/dose q6 h PO
    - IV route (intermittent)
      - Morphine 0.05–0.1 mg/kg/dose q2–4 h IV
      - Hydromorphone 0.015 mg/kg/dose q2–4 h IV
      - Fentanyl 0.5–1 mcg/kg IV q1–2 h IV
    - Patient- or caregiver-controlled analgesia
      - Patients should receive a loading dose of an analgesic before beginning PCA for maintenance
    - *Morphine*: basal rate 0–0.03 mg/kg/hour; demand dose: 0.01–0.03 mg/kg/dose (lockout every 10–15 minutes)
    - *Hydromorphone*: basal rate 0 to 0.004 mg/kg/hour; demand dose: 0.003–0.005 mg/kg/dose (lockout every 6–10 minutes)
    - There is no maximum dose of opioids. Opioids should be titrated rapidly (usually in dosage increments of 30–50% every third dose) until adequate analgesia is attained or adverse side effects develop.
  - Opioid rotation may be necessary due to tolerance, adverse side effects, or new development of hepatic or renal failure.
- Upper airway secretions (the "death rattle," pooling of secretions in the airway) occur late in the dying process and usually portend imminent death (within hours). It is not believed to cause discomfort but can be distressing to family members:
  - Non-pharmacologic interventions
    - Reposition patient
    - Minimize IV fluids
    - Reassure family members

- – Pharmacologic measures can be used although their efficacy is unclear.
  - – Glycopyrrolate 40–100 mcg/kg/dose q4–8 h
  - – Atropine (1% ophthalmic solution): 1 drop every 2–6 hours
- For patients who are DNR, laboratory testing usually is not done.

Bibliography

Komatz K, Carter B. Pain and symptom management in pediatric palliative care. *Pediatr Rev.* 2015;36(12):527–534.

Snaman JN, Baker JM, Ehrentraut JH, Anghelescu D. Pediatric oncology: Managing pain at the end of life. *Pediatr Drugs.* 2016;18:161–180.

What ChatGPT Says

Good overview but again, not much detail. ChatGPT overlaps responses relating to managing symptoms and what happens next. We have separated these steps to better parallel our own suggestions.

End-of-life care for children requires a compassionate, holistic, and family-centered approach. Diagnosing and managing end-of-life care in childhood involves a combination of medical, emotional, and supportive measures to ensure that the child's comfort and dignity are maintained. It also involves providing support to the family during this challenging time. Here are the key aspects of diagnosis and management of end-of-life care in childhood:

1. *Diagnosis and assessment*:
   a. *Recognizing end of life*: Determining when a child is approaching the end of life can be complex. Healthcare providers, including pediatricians, palliative care teams, and pediatric oncologists, will assess the child's medical condition and consider factors such as disease progression, treatment response, and overall clinical decline.
   b. *Communication*: Effective and sensitive communication with the child, parents, and caregivers is essential. The healthcare team should discuss the prognosis, goals of care, and treatment options openly, honestly, and in an age-appropriate manner.
   c. *Assessment of symptoms*: Assessing and managing the child's symptoms and distress is critical. This includes pain, shortness of breath, nausea, anxiety, and other symptoms. Symptom management may involve medications, non-pharmacological interventions, and emotional support.
2. *Management*:
   a. *Palliative care*: Pediatric palliative care is a comprehensive approach to improving the quality of life for children with life-limiting illnesses. It focuses on pain and symptom management, emotional and psychosocial support, and enhancing the child's and family's overall well-being.

b. *Hospice care*: Hospice care provides comprehensive end-of-life support, including pain and symptom management, psychosocial support, and spiritual care. Hospice services can be delivered at home, in a hospice facility, or in the hospital, depending on the family's preferences.

c. *Patient and family goals of care*: Determine and respect the child's and family's goals of care. This may include focusing on comfort, spending quality time together, and ensuring a peaceful and dignified death.

d. *Advance care planning*: Assist the family in making decisions about the child's care, such as the use of life-sustaining treatments, do-not-resuscitate (DNR) orders, and organ donation.

e. *Emotional and psychological support*: Provide emotional support to the child and family. This includes access to child life specialists, social workers, psychologists, and support groups.

f. *Spiritual and cultural support*: Respect the child's and family's spiritual and cultural beliefs and provide access to chaplains or religious leaders for spiritual guidance and support.

g. *Bereavement support*: Offer bereavement support to the family, including grief counseling and assistance with funeral planning.

h. *Practical support*: Assist the family with practical matters, such as coordinating care and arranging for respite care if needed.

i. *Comfort measures*: Focus on maintaining the child's comfort. This may include providing pain relief through medications, positioning, and comforting interventions.

j. *Continuity of care*: Ensure a smooth transition between care settings, such as from the hospital to home or hospice. This includes coordinating care and medication management.

Algorithm: Managing Symptoms at the End of Life

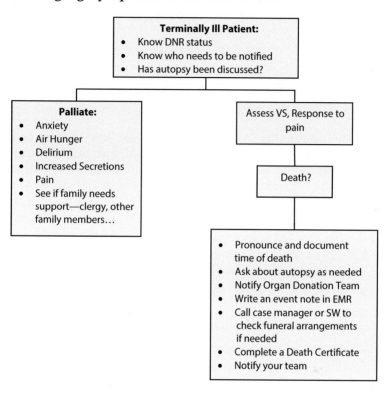

Terminally Ill Patient:
- Know DNR status
- Know who needs to be notified
- Has autopsy been discussed?

Palliate:
- Anxiety
- Air Hunger
- Delirium
- Increased Secretions
- Pain
- See if family needs support—clergy, other family members…

Assess VS, Response to pain

Death?

- Pronounce and document time of death
- Ask about autopsy as needed
- Notify Organ Donation Team
- Write an event note in EMR
- Call case manager or SW to check funeral arrangements if needed
- Complete a Death Certificate
- Notify your team

43

What To Do When a Patient Dies

- Pronounce the patient after: Assessing for pupillary reactivity, spontaneous respirations, heartbeat, pulse, and response to painful stimuli. Patients can have spontaneous respirations with very long pauses, so your assessment should take a minimum of five minutes. If all of these are absent, declare the time of death as the time you completed your exam. (Note that this does not apply to brain death which requires two physicians to independently confirm a patient's death);
- Autopsy: Unless this has been established in advance, ask the family if they are interested in an autopsy, explaining that this may help them understand the patient's death and, in a few instances, may help another family member or others.
  - This can be limited to particularly important body parts rather than a full autopsy;
  - This is done like a surgery, does not interfere with an open casket, and does not delay burial;
  - It is free;
- Organ donation: The primary care team ideally should notify the local organ procurement organization when a death is anticipated. As the on-call fellow, you may need to do that again once the patient dies (this can also be done by nursing). Do this even if you know that a patient is not a candidate for organ donation. A member of the organization, **not** you, should take the lead in approaching a potential donor/family;
- Funeral home arrangements: In some institutions, inquiring about funeral home arrangements is the responsibility of the social worker or case manager, who can also provide information and resources;
- Documentation: Write an event note in the medical record detailing the above;
- Complete a death certificate: There also may be a death certificate worksheet or electronic death certificate, autopsy request form, out-of-state burial-transit form, etc. These forms vary by state and institution. Floor nursing or admin should be able to tell you where to find these;
- Notify the primary attending and other team members of the patient's death the next day, if not already done.

DOI: 10.1201/9781003473701-47

Bibliography

Linebarger JS, Johnson V, Boss RD. Guidance for pediatric end-of-life care. *Pediatrics*. 2022;149: e2022057011.

What ChatGPT Says

Not bad, but as with other topics we believe the night-call person needs more detailed instruction, although some of this will be institution-specific. We have condensed some of the Chat suggestions and/or moved them to the prior section.

Losing a child is an incredibly painful experience, and there's no one-size-fits-all approach to grief. Every family and individual will cope differently, and it's essential to allow space for the unique ways that grief manifests. Providing emotional support, understanding, and a sense of community can be invaluable during this challenging time.

Here are steps to consider when a child dies:

1. *Allow time with the child*: It's important to allow family members and loved ones to spend time with the child, say their goodbyes, and grieve in their own way. If possible, consider allowing the child to stay with the family for a while.

2. *Support for parents and siblings*: Parents and siblings will need immediate emotional support. Allow them to grieve openly and express their feelings.

3. *Legal requirements*: Contact the appropriate authorities to initiate the necessary legal procedures, including obtaining a death certificate and arranging for an autopsy if needed.

4. *Grief counseling and support*: Seek professional grief counseling for the family members, especially parents and siblings. Grief support groups and individual counseling can help navigate the intense emotional pain. Parents will need immediate emotional support. Allow them to grieve openly and express their feelings. Siblings of the deceased child may need special attention and support. Recognize their grief and provide opportunities for them to express their feelings and ask questions.

44

What ChatGPT Has to Say: Postscript

"ChatGPT is scary good. We are not far from dangerously strong AI."—

Elon Musk

"ChatGPT is incredibly limited but good enough at some things to create a misleading impression of greatness. It's a mistake to be relying on it for anything important right now. It's a preview of progress."—

Sam Altman

We hope this manual is of some help. Since the premise is that on-call nights are so busy that young pediatric hematologist-oncologists need a digest of "How-Tos," you probably didn't have the time to read the introduction and probably won't read this chapter either. On the off chance that you, respectively, did and will, you will remember that one of our goals was to explore the usefulness of artificial intelligence in the setting of acute care PHO. We actually did ask ChatGPT "How do you manage" and "How do you evaluate" each of the chapter headings in this book. We have included the answers as part of each chapter.

What we found partly agrees with Mr. Musk ("ChatGTP is scary...") and more fully agrees with Mr. Altman. ChatGPT was not bad for a few topics (Paraspinal Mass, Differentiation Syndrome, PRES, Hemolytic Anemia, Transfusion Emergencies, Splenic Sequestration, HLH, KMP, Managing Symptoms at the End of Life, What To Do When a Patient Dies); was incomplete for most (High WBC, Hepatomegaly, Tumor Lysis Syndrome, High-Risk Fevers, Typhlitis, Severe Anemia, Thrombotic Microangiopathy, Sickle Cell Emergencies, DVTs); and had nothing or almost nothing to say about some topics (Mediastinal Masses, Methotrexate Toxicity, Arterial Strokes, Thrombocytopenia, Hemophilia, Other Factor Deficiencies, COVID Emergencies, Neonatal Hematologic Emergencies, Vascular Anomalies).

Overall, we had to conclude that at this time ChatGPT rarely added anything to our bulleted recommendations and was inaccurate or incomplete enough on other topics for us to argue that its use may not be appropriate for now. On the other hand, we share the view that AI has an impressive ability to learn and the possibility to create better management plans in the future. It just isn't there yet. An unanticipated benefit of the ChatGPT responses for trainees who may be less familiar with some of these complex topics is that it may give them more simple language with which to help explain what is going on to a family. Something to support both Mr. Musk's and Mr. Altman's views, and they are both still welcome to subsidize our future efforts.

DOI: 10.1201/9781003473701-48

Index

Note: **bold** = table, *italics* = figure

Printed in the United States
by Baker & Taylor Publisher Services